Healing Oils

Healing Oils

500 FORMULAS FOR AROMATHERAPY

Carol Schiller & David Schiller

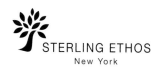

STERLING ETHOS

New York

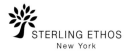

STERLING ETHOS
New York

An Imprint of Sterling Publishing Co., Inc.
1166 Avenue of the Americas
New York, NY 10036

This Sterling Ethos edition published in 2016

This publication includes alternative therapies and is intended for informational purposes only. The publisher does not claim that this publication shall provide or guarantee any benefits, healing, cure, or any results in any respect. This publication is not intended to provide or replace conventional medical advice, treatment, or diagnosis or be a substitute to consulting with a physician or other licensed medical or health-care provider. The publisher shall not be liable or responsible in any respect for any use or application of any content contained in this publication or any adverse effects, consequence, loss, or damage of any type resulting or arising from, directly or indirectly, the use or application of any content contained in this publication. Any trademarks are the property of their respective owners, are used for editorial purposes only, and the publisher makes no claim of ownership and shall acquire no right, title, or interest in such trademarks by virtue of this publication.

ISBN 978-1-4549-1776-2

Distributed in Canada by Sterling Publishing Co., Inc.
c/o Canadian Manda Group, 664 Annette Street
Toronto, Ontario, Canada M6S 2C8
Distributed in the United Kingdom by GMC Distribution Services
Castle Place, 166 High Street, Lewes, East Sussex, England BN7 1XU
Distributed in Australia by NewSouth Books
45 Beach Street, Coogee, NSW 2034, Australia

For information about custom editions, special sales, and premium and corporate purchases, please contact Sterling Special Sales at 800-805-5489 or specialsales@sterlingpublishing.com.

Manufactured in the United States of America

4 6 8 10 9 7 5 3

www.sterlingpublishing.com

Design by Rich Hazelton
Photo credits are on page 189

Dedicated to our treasured readers and to the natural therapists, practitioners, herbalists, and teachers who educate and practice from the goodness of their hearts to help alleviate discomfort and suffering, and who help guide people to live healthier, better lives. It is you who make a positive difference in this world. May you continue to do your great work.

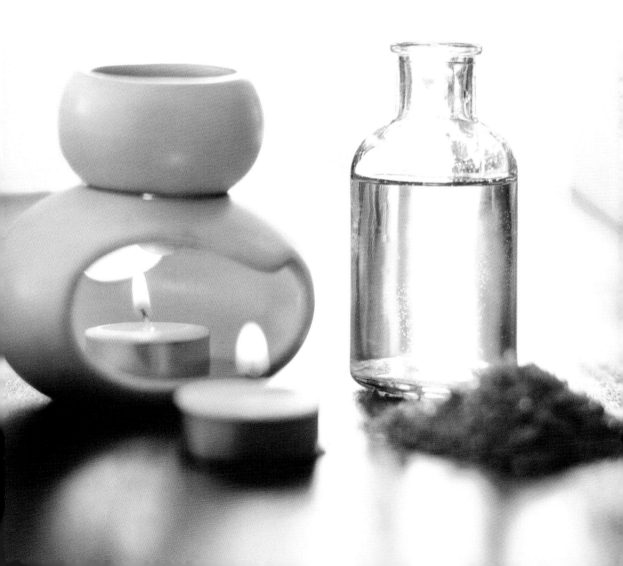

Contents

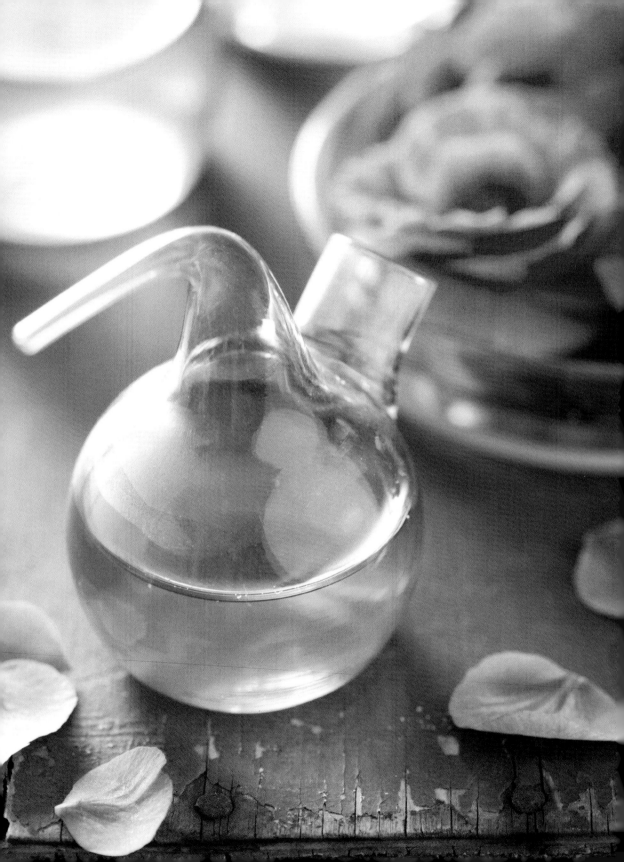

Acknowledgments

We would like to thank the following people and institutions:

Dr. Karl-Werner Quirin, co-founder and president of Flavex, a high-quality producer of CO_2 extracts in Germany. The information on the CO_2 extraction process was provided courtesy of Dr. Quirin.

Stephen Pisano, Executive Vice President and Head of Purchasing for Organic Essential Oils, at Citrus and Allied Essences, one of the most respected and high-integrity companies in the essential oil industry.

In remembrance of Sheila Anne Barry, who was the Acquisitions Director at Sterling Publishing Co. We were so lucky to have known her. If Sheila liked you, you couldn't have had a better friend than she was.

Charles Nurnberg, the former head of Sterling Publishing Co. Charlie's great efforts played a major role in the success of Sterling. It was an exciting experience to write books for him. We are thankful for all the good he did and the opportunity he gave us.

A grateful thank you to John Woodside, the former Editorial Director at Sterling Publishing, and his assistant, Emma Gonzalez. Emma was always so helpful to us. We appreciated both John and Emma very much.

Kate Zimmermann and Marilyn Kretzer, editorial department at Sterling Publishing Co.

Sharon Muir, for promoting the education of aromatherapy so that many people can learn and incorporate the essential oils into their lives. Your service has been great.

Jeffrey Schiller, for his excellent ideas.

Olivia Templeton, Lisa Lewis, Deniece May, Amy Goff, and Elizabeth Gush, for their invaluable support of the education of aromatherapy.

The public libraries, for their exceptional service. They are the greatest institutions for learning and are a vital asset to every community, providing enormous opportunities for those seeking to further their knowledge. Libraries serve as an invaluable resource of information, helping people become more informed and educated, which is vitally necessary in maintaining a free society. We commend the following individuals and express our sincere appreciation for the helpful, caring, and unsurpassed service they provide at the Phoenix Public Library: Judy De Bolt, Caren Lumley, Alicia Martin, Katie Tay, Pat Brieaddy, Bill Smith, Rob Hardin, Brandi Anton, Catherine McClarin, and David Hunt.

Amy Dodd, Judy Fleming, and Megan Jimenez, at the Glendale Community College library, who do an outstanding job every day. They are very special people.

Plant oils are a precious gift to us. We wish to express our gratitude to the people who toil the soil, sow the seeds, help the plants to grow, harvest the materials, and produce the oils. We thank as well, the people who provide the transportation for the products and the high-integrity businesses that offer these life-enhancing substances for people to greatly benefit from.

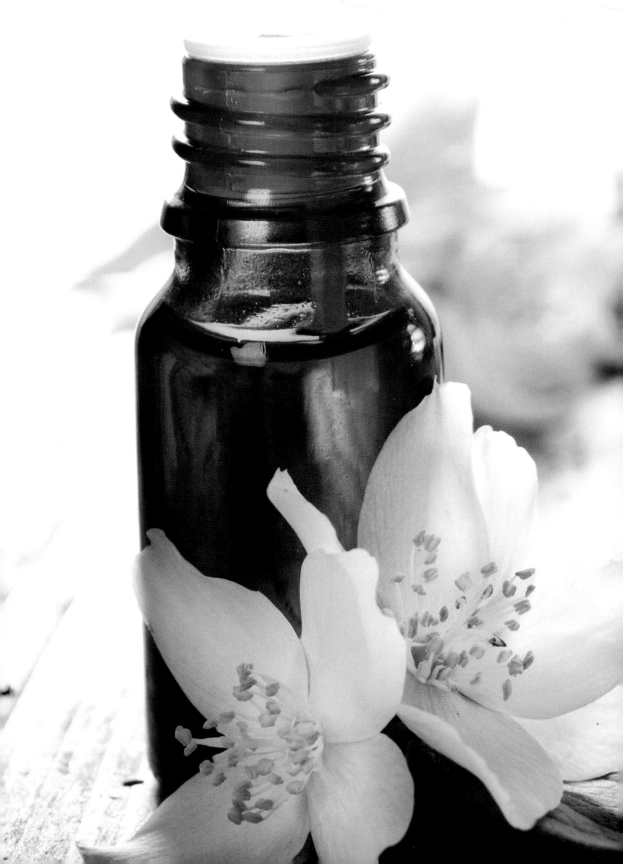

Introduction:
A GIFT FROM NATURE

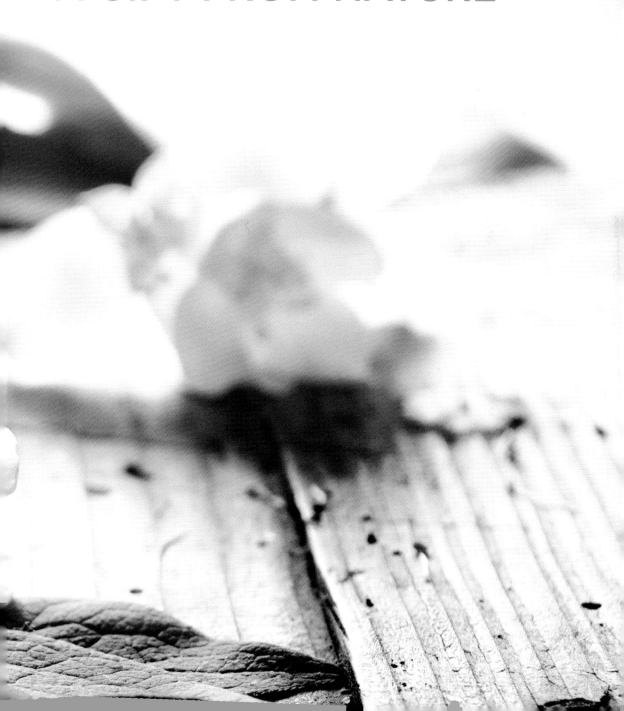

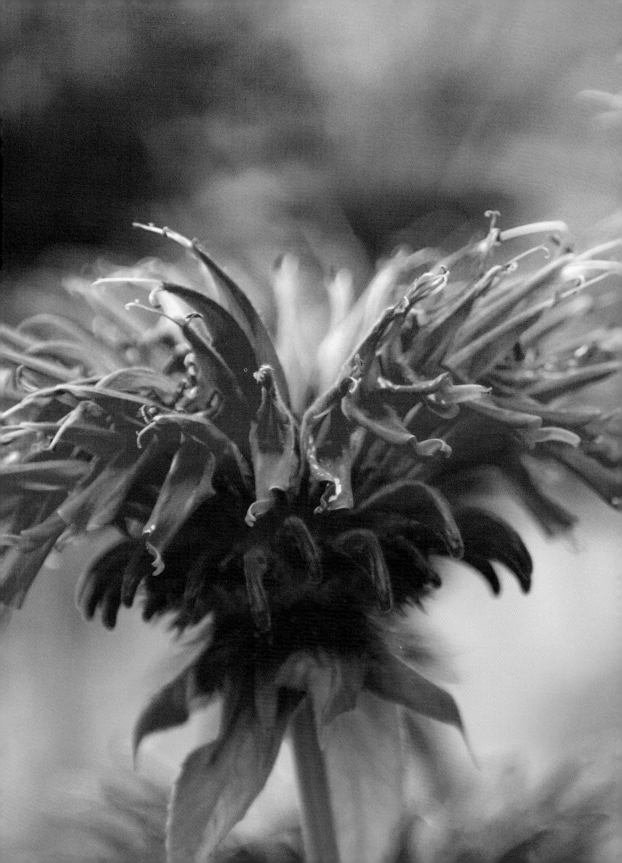

The brilliant colors of fragrant flowers, the energizing air from towering trees, and the house plants that purify our indoor air are just a few examples of nature's myriad benefits. But this is not all: plants do not only provide beauty and fresh air, they are necessary for our very existence. Without them, we would perish—lacking food to eat and oxygen to breathe.

Humans have always depended on a close relationship with nature. In order to survive, it was important to have an extensive knowledge of plant life in their immediate area to obtain food, medicine, clothing, and shelter. Humans have also discovered plant uses from close observation of animals. Sick sheep eat yarrow, lizards eat chamomile to relieve snakebites, cats and dogs chew grass to rid themselves of stomach problems, and bears eat bear's garlic as a spring tonic after awakening from hibernation. The instincts of animals to derive benefits from plants is one of the most fascinating aspects of nature.

Archaeological evidence found in Shanidar, Iraq, in 1975 indicates that Neanderthals used plants for food and medicine over 60,000 years ago. Discovered beside the ancient skeletal remains was pollen from eight species of medicinal plants, seven of which are still grown and used by Iraqi peasants today. The Ebers Papyrus, written by the Egyptians around 1550 BC, contains 877 prescriptions using medicinal plants.

Most populations in the Western world are concentrated in large cities today. Except for an occasional visit to a suburb or forest area, people live in an environment devoid of nature. While an urban lifestyle may be practical in economic terms, it can be disastrous for human health and well-being. As ailments caused by pollution and stress continue to rise annually, many people have turned to nature's herbs and essential oils to help reverse the harmful effects of urban life.

Essential oils are extracted from plants, shrubs, trees, flowers, seeds, roots, and grasses. These oils contain the essential life force of the plants. Aromatic oils promote plant growth, aid in reproduction by attracting pollinating insects, repel predators, and protect against disease. When we blend these wonderful, pure, and fragrant oils, they create the most enjoyable and effective products imaginable. The essences can be used for massage, skin and hair care, and as deodorants to keep fresh all day. When the oils are diffused or misted into the air, they produce an aroma that can smell like the perfume of a beautiful flower garden or the clean, fresh, invigorating air of a pine forest. You can also surrender yourself to the pleasures of relaxation and tranquility in a bath, foot bath, Jacuzzi, sauna, or steam room. In addition, you can treat yourself and your loved ones to a naturally fragrant home with scented candles, closets, drawers, laundry, carpets, and potpourri. Perhaps you would like to enjoy the outdoors without the fear of sunburning; carrier oils, such as jojoba, can help moisturize and protect your skin. Whatever formula you choose from this book, you will appreciate its use.

Those who use aromatic oils regularly hold them in high esteem. One can only respect the ability of essential oils to perform effectively, not just physically, but emotionally and spiritually. Even though these oils cannot completely substitute for interaction with nature, we can derive enormous benefits from their use. And they can relieve the unnatural experience of a city life that's divorced from trees, flowers, and plants.

Carol Schiller and David Schiller

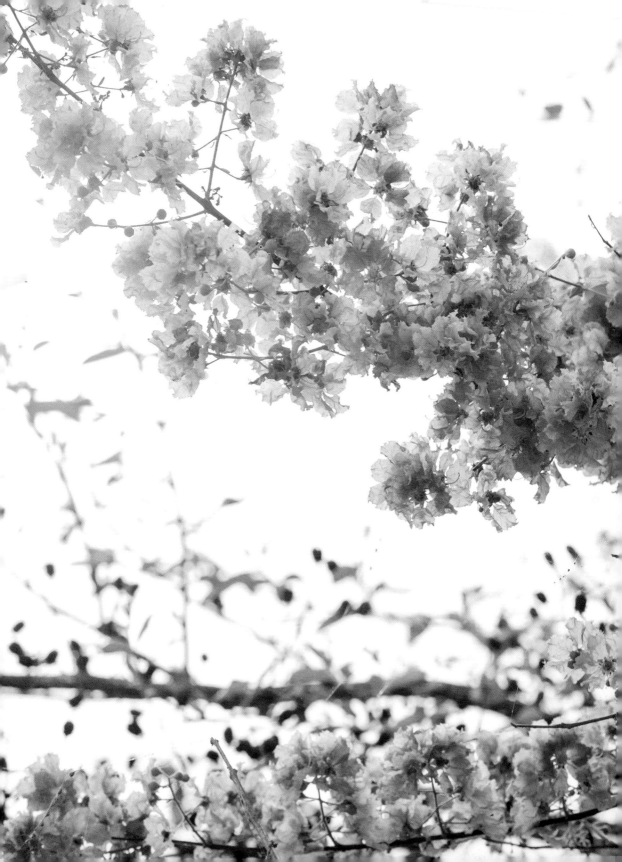

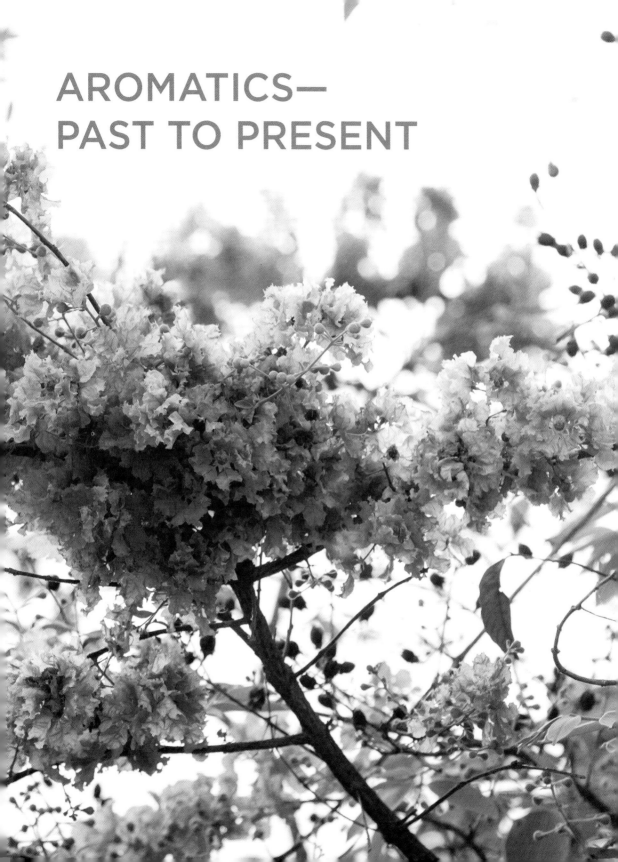

AROMATICS—
PAST TO PRESENT

The use of aromatic plants predates written records. Archaeological evidence indicates that the ancient civilizations of Egypt, Sumeria, Babylonia, Assyria, Crete, and China were skilled in extracting and blending plant oils and used ointments, fragrances, and incense. Aromatic plants were also used as medicinal remedies, and fragrant resins, gums, and woods were burned as incense during religious ceremonies as an offering for the gods.

Aromatics have been found in the tombs of Egyptian pharaohs, who lived more than 3,000 years ago. Ancient Egyptians soaked fragrant woods and resins in water and oil, then rubbed their bodies with the liquid. They also used these liquids to embalm the dead. Affluent women were so enthralled with the use of perfumes that they applied a different scent to each part of their bodies daily. Cleopatra, Egypt's famous queen, was a fragrance fanatic. She drenched the sails of her ship with perfumes to attract Mark Anthony.

The Greeks learned about the use of aromatics from the Egyptians. Greek athletes anointed themselves with fragrant oils to increase their strength for competitive games. After the Romans conquered Greece, they took full advantage of the many uses of aromatic oils as fragrances. They lavishly doused their bodies with perfume, scented their clothing, furniture, flags, military banners, and even the large amphitheatres. Roman soldiers were anointed with perfumes before battle. At one of Nero's feasts, a guest was asphyxiated by showers of rose fragrance. In the 1st century, Rome received between 2,500 and 3,000 tons of frankincense, and between 450 and 600 tons of myrrh from Arabia.

The fall of the Western Roman Empire brought an abrupt but temporary halt to the most extravagant use of aromatics ever seen. The city of Constantinople then became an important center of civilization, and its citizens in turn used aromatics lavishly. Overindulgence in fragrances by the general populace infuriated the Church, however. Perfume use became synonymous with degeneracy and immorality, and the early Church condemned the personal use of aromatics. Consequently, widespread use of plant oils ended in Europe. However, plant oil use continued in the Middle East and Far East.

In the 7th century, the Arabs continued the traditional art of perfumery and played an important role in introducing perfumes to other parts of the world. During the 10th century, Avicenna, an Arabian scientist, discovered the distillation process for extracting essences from plants and flowers. In the 13th century, the gallant knights and crusaders brought back scented gifts to Europe. As new trade routes to China and India opened. Europeans rekindled their passion for fragrance.

During the 14th century, the Black Death ravaged Europe and Asia, claiming millions of lives. The aromatic plants clove, cypress, cedar, pine, sage, rosemary, and thyme were burned in the streets, hospitals, and sickrooms in an attempt to ward off the infectious disease. Perfumers and those who were in daily contact with aromatic plants seemed immune to the plague.

The use of herbology and aromatics increased in popularity during the onset of yet another plague in Europe in 1665. It was recommended that every home burn aromatic substances to disinfect the air against the deadly bacteria. Aromatics reached another peak in 18th century France, during the reign of Louis XV. On festive occasions, even the water in Parisian fountains was perfumed. In his palace, various perfumes were used daily.

In the mid-19th century, scientists began producing synthetic versions of essential plant oils, replacing these pure and precious natural oils that have been treasures for centuries.

Synthetic scents and fragrances are usually produced from petroleum derivatives and other synthetic materials. They not only pose harmful side effects for individuals using them, but processing these chemicals also pollutes the earth, water, and air. Essential oils, on the other hand, help balance the human body and work in harmony with nature. The use of these natural oils has gained popularity as more people become aware of their remarkable benefits. If we can use history as a guide to the future, perhaps people will rediscover what ancient people knew so well—the important value of plants and their valuable oils.

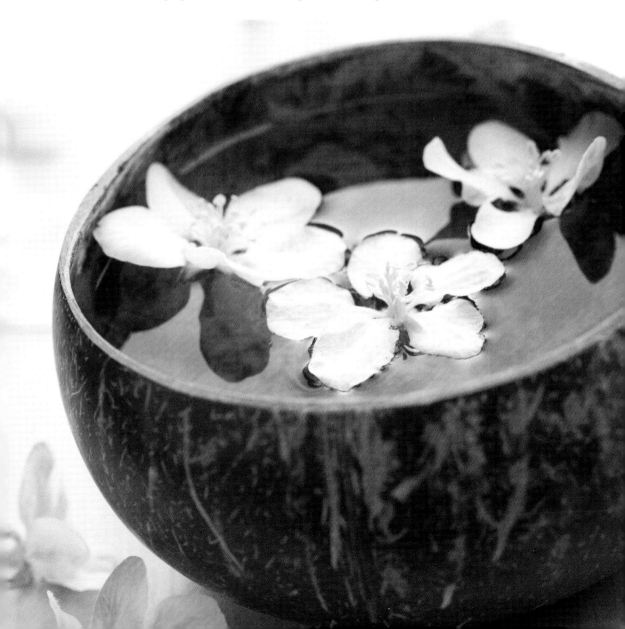

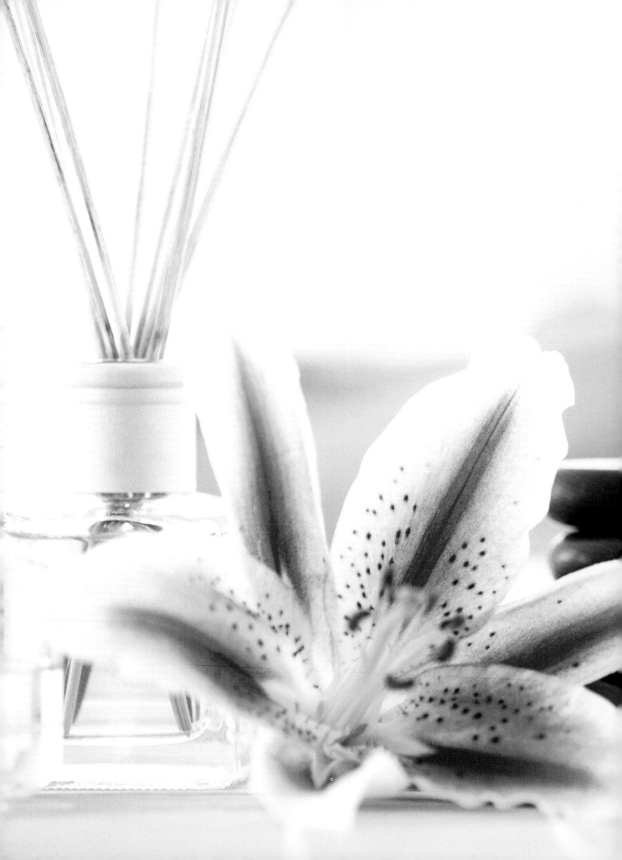

Combining Scent and Touch

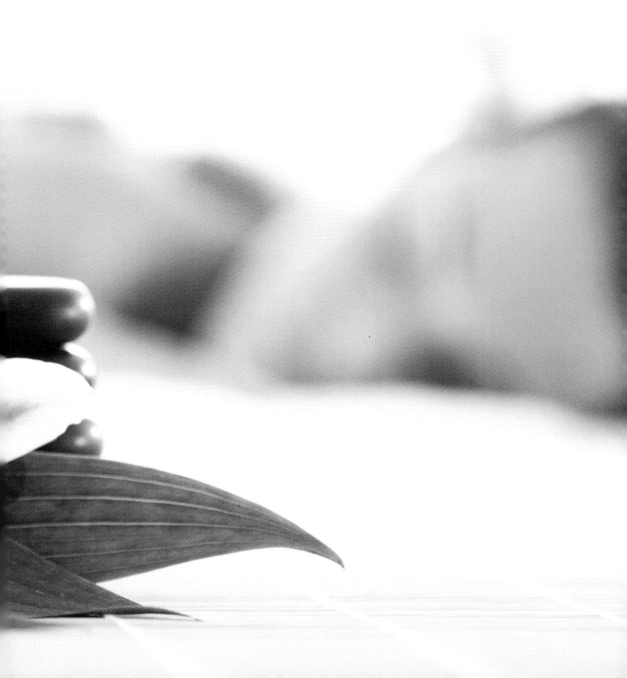

The Sense of Smell

We think of the nose as primarily an organ of smell. However, its main function is moderating the temperature of inhaled air, which protects the linings of the lungs. Secondarily, the nose serves as a conduit that guides scent into the olfactory system. But only about 2 percent of inhaled air reaches the olfactory epithelium, which consists of two patches of tissue, covering an area of 1 square inch (2.5 square cm), in the upper rear of the nasal cavities. This is where we detect smell.

The olfactory nerve contains about 50 million smell receptors that protrude from mucous membranes. These hairs collect odors and convert them into messages which are relayed to the olfactory nerve and then to the brain for processing. Olfactory cells are the only nerve cells that are regenerated in the body.

Smell signals travel through the limbic system and play an important role in provoking feelings and memories. Among the structures that form the limbic system are the amygdala, where we process anger; the septum pellucidum, where we process pleasurable sensations; and the hippocampus, which regulates how much attention we give these emotions and memories.

Since the sense of smell has a powerful impact on memory, odor can evoke the recall of emotions. The subconscious mind stores our memories of past experiences in a memory bank. When inhaling an

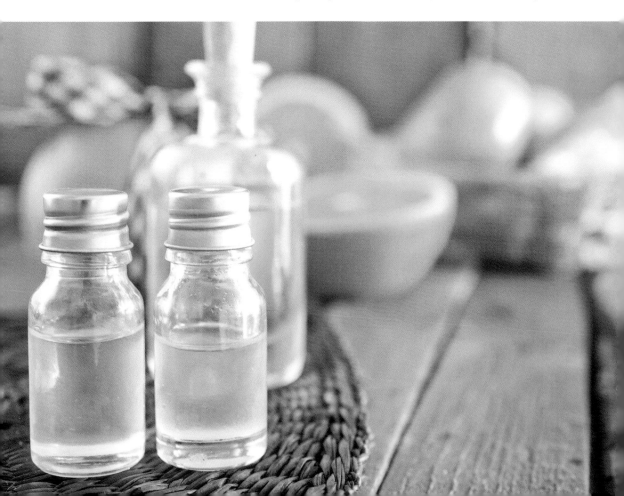

aroma, the olfactory cells transmit a direct signal to the brain's memory bank. As this process occurs, a particular memory may be activated. If the scent is recognized, it may trigger a memory of past events and emotions associated with that particular odor. The smell memory may also trigger changes in body temperature, appetite, stress level, and sexual arousal. This close connection between smell and memory may help determine why certain individuals prefer one scent to another.

The chemical substances in scent that affect reproductive behavior and act as a sexual excitant are known as *pheromones*. Pheromones are present in perspiration, saliva, vaginal secretions and urine. The apocrine glands, mainly located in the armpits and around the groin, produce pheromones. These glands are largest during a person's reproducing years. Secretions from the apocrine glands are odorless, however; odor occurs only after bacteria present react to the perspiration.

In one study, perspiration collected from men's underarms was swabbed three times a week on the upper lips of women whose menstrual cycles were less than 26 days or more than 33 days. After 3 months, all the women's cycles were regulated to 29.5 days—the optimum length for maximizing fertility. Menstrual cycles of women who live or work together become synchronized over a period of time. Many have speculated that this is due to a woman being exposed to another woman's perspiration (smelled over several months) and then adapting to the other woman's cycle. Men who are around women have more rapid hair growth, and women who are around men have more regulated cycles. Women are particularly sensitive to the odor of pheromones just before ovulation—about 1,000 times more so than at any other time during their cycle.

The most acute sense of smell known is that of the Chinese emperor moth, which can detect a scent it recognizes over 6 miles away. The male silkworm moth comes in a distant second, with its ability to detect the odor of the female silkworm's sexual secretion over 2 miles away. Although smell is not a highly developed human sense, smell remains nearly 10,000 times more sensitive than taste. Dogs are estimated to be over 1 million times more odor-sensitive than humans.

The connection between sex and scent in humans seems less important than it does for insects and animals. The pheromones that send an insect into a rage of passion do not affect humans the same way. Comparatively, humans do not demonstrate as intense or impulsive a response to scent signals from the opposite sex. Rats in the laboratory deprived of their sense of smell from birth, have low levels of growth hormones produced by the pituitary gland. Their growth is stunted and their testicles are subnormal. One out of 4 people who suffer from *anosmia* (loss or impairment of the sense of smell) lose interest in sexual activity. Hamsters that cannot smell their mates entirely lose interest in them.

Anosmia affects 2 million people in the United States. *Parosmia* is a common abnormality that causes a distorted sense of smell. The perception of a given scent may be interpreted as a consistent bad smell, similar to fecal matter. Both conditions, anosmia and parosmia, can result from head injuries or diseases.

Today, in our eagerness to deodorize our bodies and make them fragrant, we have disguised our natural odor communication. Nevertheless, we still communicate through our natural scents, but to a lesser extent. To achieve a richer life, we must develop greater understanding of how scents affect our health and behavior. Only then will we begin to appreciate this most invaluable sense and become more conscious of its myriad messages.

The Sense of Touch

Touch is a very important part of life. It is a language that communicates love, understanding, and reassurance and at the same time creates a comforting and healing effect. Many of us go through life being "touch starved" and rarely experience the wonderful feeling of being fully satisfied. Research in recent years has revealed that deprivation of touch can lead not only to emotional disturbance, but also to diminished intellectual ability, impaired physical growth, reduced sexual interest and deterioration of the immune system. In addition, many forms of deviant behavior, such as those involving depression violence, aggression, and hyperactivity have been traced to the lack of touch.

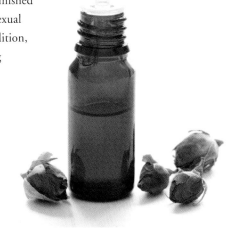

In a study conducted at the University of Wisconsin, baby monkeys deprived of their mother's bodily comfort grew up to be irritable, aggressive, and violent. When orphaned human babies have experienced deprivation of touch in orphanages, many wasted away and died of malnutrition. Newly born animals not licked by the mother shortly after birth usually die.

Massage

For thousands of years, massage has been used as a therapeutic tool to nurture and heal the body. In Greece in the early 5th century BC, Hippocrates, the father of medicine, wrote about the benefits of massage. Asclepiades, an ancient Greek physician, challenged current medical thought after learning the value of massage and relied exclusively upon its use to restore and maintain health. The renowned Roman naturalist Pliny found relief from chronic asthma by having his body rubbed regularly. Julius Caesar was pinched daily all over his body to ease nerve pain and headaches from epilepsy.

During the Middle Ages, massage was almost forgotten until the French physician Ambroise Paré revived the art in the 16th century.

In the early 19th century, Per Henrik Ling, a Swedish fencing master and gymnastics instructor, used the massage technique *percussion* to overcome rheumatism. Recognizing the healing potential of massage, Ling combined its use with his teachings. Ling's efforts and dedication gained him official recognition, and in 1813 the Royal Gymnastic Central Institute, in Stockholm, sponsored by the Swedish government, included massage in its curriculum. After Ling's death in 1839, his former students published his work on massage. Massage gained popularity, thereafter, and institutes and spas opened in Germany, Austria, and France offering this therapy. This was the beginning of what is now known as Swedish massage.

In the United Sates, it wasn't until the early 1970s that people other than dancers, athletes, and members of spas and health clubs were aware of the benefits of massage. Massage is widely recognized today for its therapeutic value, and the practice continues to flourish in the Western World.

The Importance of Massage

The epidermis (outer lay of skin) and the layers beneath are designed to process sensation. Feeling is transmitted to the body and brain through an elaborate network of touch receptors to form natural electrical charges. The skin's sensitivity as well as its ability to relay tactile messages is why massage can improve gland, organ, and nerve function, while relaxing muscles and producing a positive emotional feeling. When touch, in the form of massage, is combined with essential oils, the results can be wonderful.

Preparing for a Massage

Be sure to avoid wounded areas and exercise special caution with pregnant women. To make massage more enjoyable, please follow these guidelines.

- The room for the massage should be comfortable, quiet, and warm, and provide a retreat from worldly stress and tensions.

- Continual concentration is necessary while giving a massage; therefore, chattering should be discouraged.

- Some people prefer to relax with soft music in the background.

- A soft, thick cushion draped with a towel or sheet may be used if a massage table is unavailable. If the massage is given on the floor, padding should extend beyond the person's body.

- Add a pleasant essential oil fragrance to the room before the treatment.

- Keep extra towels, blankets, and oil nearby to avoid searching for them during the treatment.

- Hands should be clean and warm before beginning the massage. Cold hands on a warm back are very uncomfortable and could make the body tense.

- Remove all jewelry.

- Wear comfortable, loose clothing.

- Warm the carrier oil (see massage oil section) that will be used by placing the container in warm water or near a heater. Pour a small amount into your palm, and rub both hands together until warmth is generated. Then massage the oil into the skin.

- Drop the essential oils over the carrier oil. Massage into the specific areas according to the instructions for the formula being used.

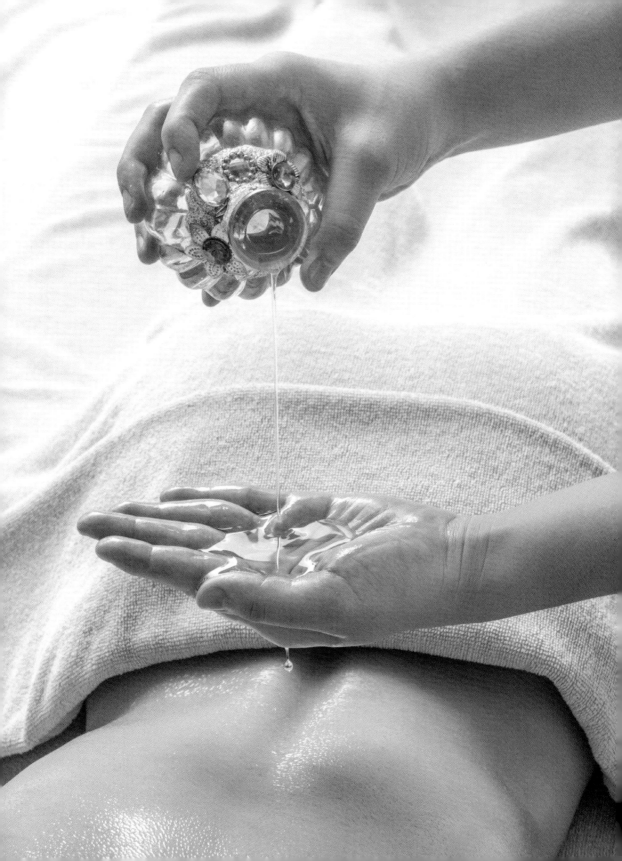

- It is important to feel relaxed while giving the massage, since tension can be transmitted to the person receiving the massage.

- If possible, maintain constant touch by gently resting one hand on the person receiving the massage when you move to a different position or side.

- Wash your hands at the end of the session.

Massage Therapies and Techniques

Swedish Massage

Stroke Movements: Slow, deliberate, continuous sequence, flowing.

Benefits: Relaxing, relieves stress and tension, tones the muscles, improves circulation and lymph flow, and gives the mind and body an overall sense of well-being.

Oils: Choose an aromatherapy massage formula listed in the Aromatherapy Formulas chapter. In order to grasp the muscles properly, the oil should be applied gradually throughout the treatment.

❁   ❁   ❁

Massage Techniques

Step 1, Gliding Stroke: Gently glide both hands over the skin, using long, broad, smooth strokes. Use this technique at the beginning and end of the treatment to relax the body. Whether you apply gentle or deep pressure depends on the person's preference and tolerance of pain.

Step 2, Muscle Kneading: Use both hands alternately to grasp, lift, and gently squeeze the muscles in a continuous kneading motion, keeping your hands on the body at all times. The amount of pressure applied can be determined by the depth of penetration needed and the receiver's pain tolerance. Kneading movements should always be in the direction of the heart. This technique helps relax and tone the muscles.

Step 3, Deep Tissue Pressure: Use the thumbs, fingertips, or heels of the hands to work deeper into the muscles and around the joints. With the fingertips or ball of each thumb, gradually press deeply into the muscle, using small, circular movements. It is important that you move the underlying tissue and do not slide your fingers across the skin. Avoid applying pressure on bony areas, such as the spine and rib cage.

Percussion: This form of massage includes hacking, beating, and cupping. It may be used on soft tissue areas, such as the back (avoiding the spine), thighs, and buttocks. These strokes stimulate the body, break up congestion, and tone the muscles. As you begin a different stroke, maintain the same rhythm.

Hacking: With the outside edge of both hands, alternately create a chopping motion directly on the muscles.

Beating: With loosely clenched fists, alternately "beat" the muscles, using the fleshy side of the hand.

Cupping: With your palms in a cupped position and the fingers held together, alternately "slap" the muscle area, which will create a loud sound.

Reflexology

Stroke Movements: Slow.

Benefits: Relaxing, relieves stress and tension, and revitalizes the body.

Oils: Choose an aromatherapy massage formula, especially from the foot or hand rejuvenation category in the Aromatherapy Formulas chapter.

Powder: For a dry massage, without oils, choose a foot powder from the formula section.

❋　❋　❋

Reflexology Techniques

Massage the entire hand or foot to encourage muscle relaxation. When the person becomes relaxed, apply direct and circular pressure alternately.

Direct Pressure: Pinpoint a painful area using your thumb or fingertip. Gently apply pressure directly on the sensitive point and hold your thumb or finger down firmly for several seconds. Release, then reapply pressure again. As you repeat this technique, gradually increase the amount of pressure according to the person's pain tolerance.

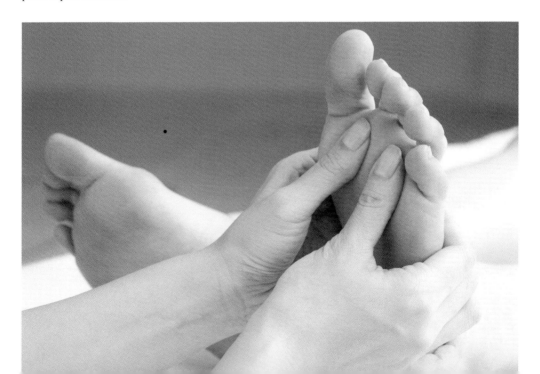

Circular Pressure: Slowly rotate your thumb or fingertip in a circular motion over the entire foot. As you find painful areas, press down firmly into the spot and manipulate the reflex point with circular movements. Gradually increase the amount of pressure according to the person's pain tolerance.

Caution: Do not use reflexology on a pregnant woman. Certain reflex points can trigger the onset of childbirth.

Massage Formulas for Restlessness

Massage one of these formulas into the abdomen, neck, and shoulders. Please read the Safety Guidelines and Helpful Hints section before using.

palmarosa	5 drops
petitgrain	4 drops
neroli	3 drops
sandalwood	3 drops
carrier oil	1 tablespoon (15 ml)

dill	4 drops
vetiver	4 drops
marjoram	4 drops
anise	3 drops
carrier oil	1 tablespoon (15 ml)

spikenard	5 drops
marjoram	4 drops
ylang-ylang	3 drops
anise	3 drops
carrier oil	1 tablespoon (15 ml)

vetiver	5 drops
lavender	5 drops
celery	3 drops
mandarin	2 drops
carrier oil	1 tablespoon (15 ml)

vetiver	5 drops
marjoram	5 drops
guaiacwood	3 drops
celery	2 drops
carrier oil	1 tablespoon (15 ml)

mandarin	5 drops
vetiver	5 drops
dill	5 drops
carrier oil	1 tablespoon (15 ml)

guaiacwood	5 drops
marjoram	4 drops
dill	4 drops
mandarin	2 drops
carrier oil	1 tablespoon (15 ml)

guaiacwood	5 drops
champaca flower	4 drops
anise	3 drops
coriander	3 drops
carrier oil	1 tablespoon (15 ml)

Massage to Soothe Abdominal Discomfort

Massage one of these formulas on the abdominal area to relieve pressure, cramps, and/or other discomfort. Please read the Safety Guidelines and Helpful Hints section before using.

spikenard	5 drops
fennel	4 drops
caraway	4 drops
lemon	2 drops
carrier oil	1 tablespoon (15 ml)

vetiver	5 drops
cardamom	4 drops
lemongrass	3 drops
anise	3 drops
carrier oil	1 tablespoon (15 ml)

sweet basil	4 drops
lemon	4 drops
anise	4 drops
ginger	3 drops
carrier oil	1 tablespoon (15 ml)

spearmint	5 drops
cardamom	4 drops
fennel	3 drops
spikenard	3 drops
carrier oil	1 tablespoon (15 ml)

lemon	4 drops		peppermint	5 drops
chamomile	4 drops		vetiver	4 drops
guaiacwood	4 drops		ginger	3 drops
sandalwood	3 drops		lemongrass	3 drops
carrier oil	1 tablespoon (15 ml)		carrier oil	1 tablespoon (15 ml)

vetiver	5 drops		bois de rose	4 drops
celery	4 drops		celery	3 drops
peppermint	4 drops		lemongrass	3 drops
caraway	2 drops		juniper berries	3 drops
carrier oil	1 tablespoon (15 ml)		vanilla CO_2	2 drops
			carrier oil	1 tablespoon (15 ml)

Massage to Soothe Lower Back

Many days are lost in the workplace due to people having lower back problems. Massage one of these formulas along the lower back until the oil is fully absorbed. It may be necessary to do this massage more than once a day. Please read the Safety Guidelines and Helpful Hints section before using.

vetiver	5 drops		ylang-ylang	5 drops
neroli	4 drops		black pepper	3 drops
cypress	3 drops		anise	3 drops
bois de rose	2 drops		sweet basil	3 drops
nutmeg	1 drop		nutmeg	1 drop
carrier oil	1 tablespoon (15 ml)		carrier oil	1 tablespoon (15 ml)

marjoram	4 drops
spikenard	4 drops
champaca flower	3 drops
lavender	2 drops
anise	2 drops
carrier oil	1 tablespoon (15 ml)

guaiacwood	4 drops
ylang-ylang	4 drops
juniper berries	3 drops
ginger	2 drops
vanilla CO_2	2 drops
carrier oil	1 tablespoon (15 ml)

champaca flower	5 drops
spikenard	4 drops
sage	3 drops
cardamom	2 drops
nutmeg	1 drop
carrier oil	1 tablespoon (15 ml)

ylang-ylang	3 drops
sage	3 drops
fennel	3 drops
guaiacwood	3 drops
cinnamon	3 drops
carrier oil	1 tablespoon (15 ml)

bois de rose	4 drops
caraway	4 drops
allspice	4 drops
thyme	3 drops
carrier oil	1 tablespoon (15 ml)

marjoram	5 drops
elemi	5 drops
ylang-ylang	5 drops
carrier oil	1 tablespoon (15 ml)

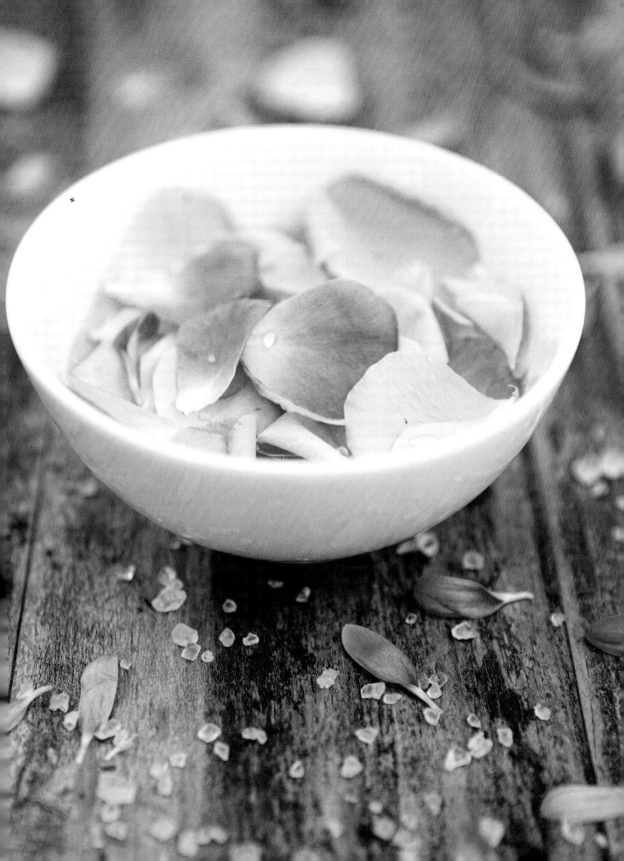

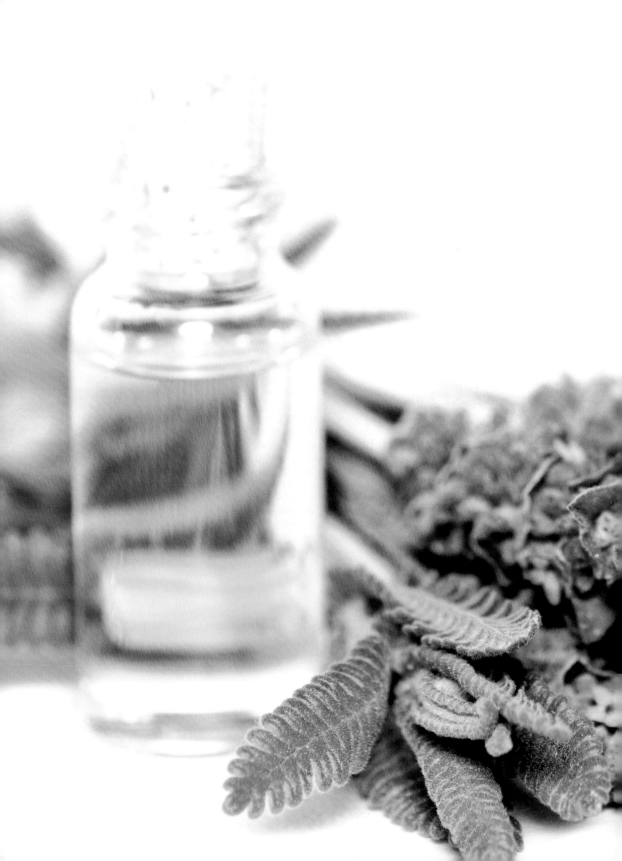

Selecting and Using Pure Oils

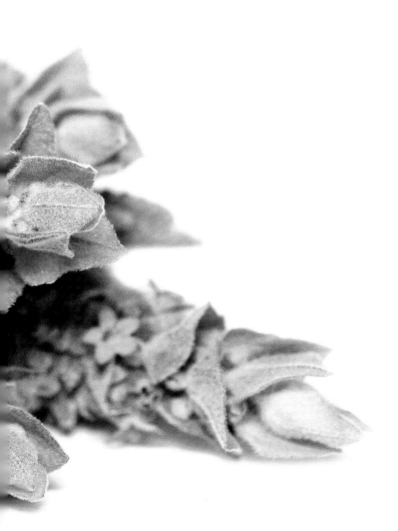

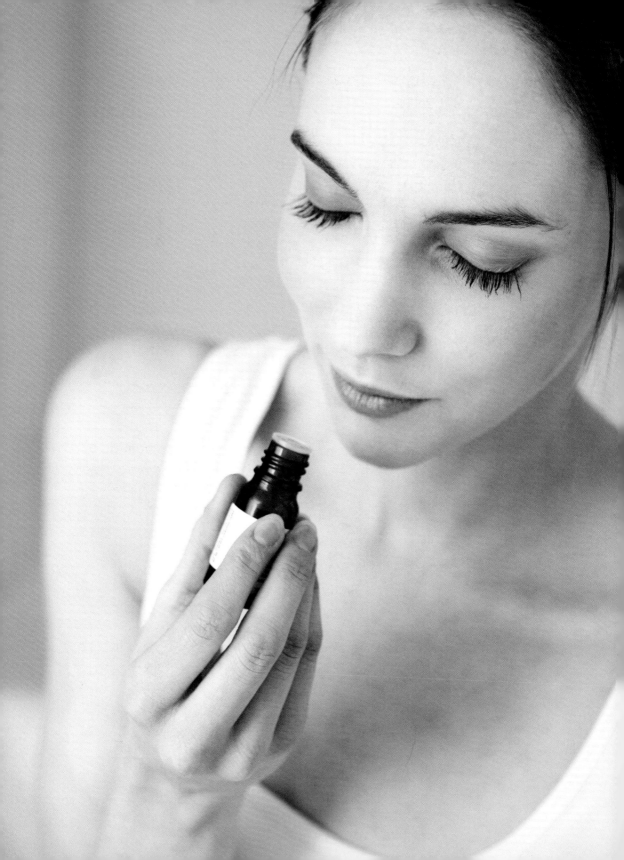

Safety Guidelines and Helpful Hints

Essential oils can be extremely beneficial when used properly; therefore, please follow these guidelines:

- The formulas in this book are for adults over 18 years old, unless stated otherwise. For children over ten years of age, reduce the number of drops to half for each formula.

- Essential oils are highly concentrated substances and should be diluted in a carrier oil such as almond (sweet), jojoba, macadamia nut, or sesame oil before being applied on the skin, in order to prevent skin irritation. If any skin irritation should occur as a result of using the essential oils, immediately apply additional carrier oil to the area. This will quickly soothe the skin. Also, dabbing on some cornstarch can be helpful.

- When applying essential oils on the skin, using a mist spray, or taking a scented bath, be careful not to get the oils into the eyes. If this should occur, flush the eyes with cool water.

- Care must be taken when using carrier and essential oils during pregnancy. Many of the oils have a stimulating effect on the uterus, which can be very helpful at the appropriate time to facilitate childbirth. However, if those oils are used prior to the time of childbirth, they can bring on premature labor. Even certain common spices, herbs, and vegetables, such as celery, carrots, parsley, basil, bay leaves, marjoram, saffron, and safflower oil can stimulate uterine contractions.

- Small amounts (two to three drops at one time) of the following essential oils are known to be safe during pregnancy: bergamot, coriander, cypress, frankincense, geranium, ginger, grapefruit, lavandin, lavender, lemon, lime, mandarin, neroli, orange, patchouli, petitgrain, sandalwood, tangelo, tangerine, tea tree, and temple orange. Sesame oil can be used as a carrier oil.

- A woman nursing her baby should exercise caution when using the essential oils as the effects of the oils will be readily passed on to the infant.

- If a person is highly allergic, a simple test can determine if there is any sensitivity to a particular oil. Rub a drop of carrier oil on the upper chest area, and, in twelve hours, check to see if there is redness or any other skin reaction. If the skin is clear, dilute one drop of an essential oil in twenty drops of the same carrier oil and again apply to the upper chest area. If there is no skin reaction after twelve hours, both the carrier and the essential oil can be used.

- Do not consume alcohol, except for a small glass of wine with a meal, in the time period when using essential oils.

- Do not use essential oils while on medication because the oils might interfere with the medicine.

- After an essential oil blend is applied on the skin, avoid, for at least four hours, sunbathing, sauna/steam room, or a hot bath, in order to prevent the possibility of skin irritation. This precaution is especially important when using phototoxic and other essential oils that can irritate the skin.

- Since the following oils tend to be irritating to the skin, take extra care when using them, especially if you have dry skin: Cinnamon, clove, grapefruit, lemon, lemongrass, lime, mandarin, melissa, orange, black pepper, peppermint, and spearmint.

- If a person has sensitive skin, the essential oils in foot and hand baths and massage oil formulas should be reduced to half strength.

- There are people with extremely sensitive skin who cannot tolerate the essential oils without experiencing skin irritation. If this is the case, discontinue use.

- The resins of benzoin, Peru balsam, and tolu balsam can be thick and sticky, and therefore difficult to use. To make them more workable, place a small piece of beeswax into a clean, empty glass baby food jar, put the jar into a pan of water, and heat on a low flame. When the wax liquefies, add the resin and an equal amount of carrier oil and stir well. Remove the jar from the heated pan and allow to cool for several minutes before adding the essential oils.

- Many essential oils will remove the finish when spilled on furniture; therefore, be careful when handling the bottles.

- Light and oxygen cause oils to deteriorate rapidly. Refrigeration does not prevent spoilage, but diminishes the speed at which it occurs. Therefore, oils should be stored in brown glass bottles in a dark and cool place.

- Always use a glass dropper when measuring drops of essential oil.

- Keep all bottles tightly closed to prevent the oils from evaporating and oxidizing.

- Always store essential oils out of sight and reach of children.

- It is important to label all bottles containing essential oil blends.

- If there is leftover oil from a massage formula, label the bottle and save for next time.

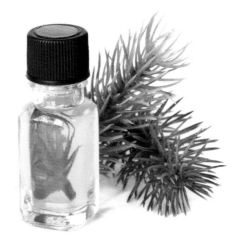

Methods of Extraction

The extraction process is a factor in determining the purity of the oil. Before purchasing carrier and essential oils, it is important to become knowledgeable of the different methods of extraction.

Steam Distillation

Steam from boiling water is used to extract the essential oil from the plant material. As the steam rises and passes through a cold coil, it turns into a liquid. The essential oil floats to the top and is skimmed off. Steam distillation is extensively used and produces a good-quality essential oil.

Carbon Dioxide (CO_2) Extraction

CO_2 extraction is the most modern extraction method available, using high pressure, and lower temperatures, than steam distillation. There are two types of oils using carbon dioxide (CO_2): one is called *Select*; the other is *Total*.

In CO_2 extraction, the plant material is placed into a chamber to which compressed CO_2 gas is released. The temperature is set to a range of 105–140°F (40–60°C). As the gas passes through the plant material, it draws out the components.

The difference between the Select and the Total processes is in the amount of pressure used. The pressure determines the density of the carbon dioxide gas and the ability of the gas to dissolve the plant material, as well as the viscosity of the oil. Select extracts are produced at 90–120 bar pressure, and the Total at 300–500 bar pressure. When the process is completed, the pressure is lowered, and the extracted components precipitate out and are collected. The CO_2 gas is then recompressed and recycled to be used again, without leaving any residue in the extracted oil.

The Select oil contains components similar to oils extracted through steam distillation. The Total method extracts a great amount of the plant components. The oil is considered more identical to the plant material it is obtained from, containing more constituents than from the Select method. The Total oils tend to be thicker, and some are semisolid. This extract is comparable in components to the hexane-solvent extracted oil. For example, when an extraction is done on the fennel plant, the Select extract consists of mainly essential oil, while the Total extract contains the essential oil together with the full amount of fatty oil (vegetal oil) that naturally occurs in the plant material.

Since the CO_2 process equipment is more costly, the extracted essential oils are more expensive than the steam distilled. However, CO_2 extracts have superior quality and composition.

Cold-Pressed Citrus Oils

Essential oils from citrus fruit require a different method of extraction. Citrus oils are produced from the citrus peel, using a cold-pressed method. The fruits are placed on a conveyor belt and then dropped into a cup with knives. As the cup closes, the knives puncture the fruit and remove the peel. The peel is then soaked in water and put through a centrifuge process to separate out the essential oil.

Maceration

Flowers such as rose, jasmine, and other plant materials are soaked in hot fatty oil until the cells rupture and the oil absorbs the aromatic essence contained in the flowers.

Solvent Extraction

The plant material is bathed in solvents such as hexane and other toxic chemicals, which are used to extract the oil. A high percentage of carrier/vegetal oils are extracted in this manner. Concretes are also obtained by using this method, which produces a semi-solid wax. Absolutes are a secondary product made from concretes. The process involves adding ethanol to dissolve the concrete, removing some of the heavy components. After the alcohol is evaporated out, a semi-heavy liquid remains, which is the absolute. Examples of plant materials commonly used for concretes and absolutes are jasmine, linden blossom, lotus, and rose.

Solvent-extracted oils are less expensive to produce than the cold-pressed, expeller-pressed, steam-distilled, and CO_2-extracted methods, and produce a higher yield. However, toxic residues remain in the oil, which makes this product undesirable for aromatherapy use.

Cold-Pressed and Expeller-Pressed Extraction of Vegetal Oils

Seeds, nuts, fruits, and vegetables are pressed without the use of high heat to preserve the components in the oil. These methods produce a quality oil.

Cold-pressed oils are produced by a mechanical batch-pressing process in which heat-producing friction is minimized, keeping temperatures below 120°F (49°C). The expeller-pressed method generates more heat to extract the oil, so in-line refrigerated cooling devices are added to the presses to keep the temperatures down to 185°F (85°C) during the pressing. A large percentage of vegetal oils are usually refined afterward using high heat and harsh chemicals that include the following:

- **Degumming:** Chlorophyll, vitamins, and minerals are removed from the oil.

- **Refining:** An alkaline solution called lye is added to refine the oil.

- **Bleaching:** Fuller's earth, a naturally occurring clay-like substance, is added as a bleaching agent and then filtered out, further removing nutritive substances. The oil at this stage becomes clear.

- **Deodorizing:** The oil is deodorized by steam distillation at high temperatures over 450°F (232°C) for 30 to 60 minutes.

- **Winterizing:** The oil is then cooled and filtered. This process prevents the oil from becoming cloudy during cold temperatures.

The finished product is nutrient deficient, with only fatty acids remaining. Therefore, it is important to check the product label on the container to ensure that the oil is unrefined, containing all the valuable nutrients.

Selecting Quality Oils

Never use synthetic oils and oils extracted by chemical solvents. Many synthetic oils on the market today replicate the fragrances of natural oils, and many people unknowingly use them, hoping to derive their benefits. The synthetic chemicals that create these products do not contain the beneficial properties of pure plant oils. In addition, many synthetic compounds can be very irritating to the body and nervous system. Oils extracted with solvents contain toxic residues harmful to the body. It is important to select *unrefined* carrier oils, and essential oils extracted by *steam distillation* or which have been *pressed mechanically* or by an *expeller*.

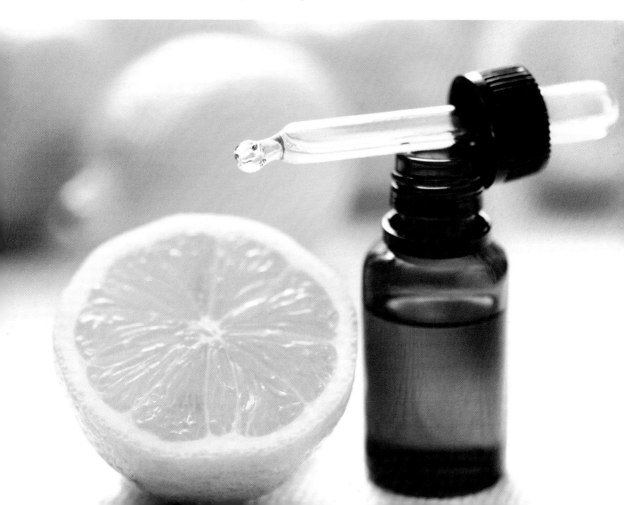

Substitutions for Oils

Many essential oils in this book are quite expensive. In order to economize in making the blends, you can substitute oils and still derive up to 90 percent of the benefits of the original formulas.

Original Oil	Substitute Oil(s)
jasmine	ylang-ylang
neroli	mandarin + petitgrain (equal parts)
chamomile	lavender
rose	bois de rose
bergamot	grapefruit
tea tree	cajeput + lavender (equal parts)
melissa	lemon + petitgrain (equal parts)
sandalwood	cedarwood
clary sage	sage + lavender (equal parts)
myrrh	myrrh oil blend
vanilla CO_2	guaiacwood

Myrrh Oil Blend: Here's an inexpensive way to make your own myrrh oil blend. Purchase myrrh resin or powder and finely grind it in a coffee mill. Then add the fine powder to a carrier oil. Heat the mixture for 30 minutes and allow to sit for a few days before using. If the blend feels gritty, filter the oil through a coffee filter.

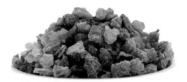
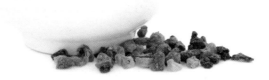

Other Substitutions

You may also substitute these essential oils for each other (lemon for lime or lime for lemon):

lemon	lime
spearmint	peppermint
mandarin	orange
grapefruit	lemon

Drop Equivalents

20 drops	=	⅛ teaspoon	=	1 ml
100 drops	=	1 teaspoon	=	5 ml
300 drops	=	1 tablespoon	=	15 ml
600 drops	=	1 ounce	=	30 ml

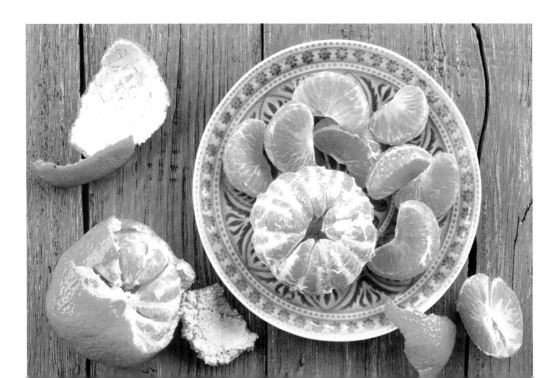

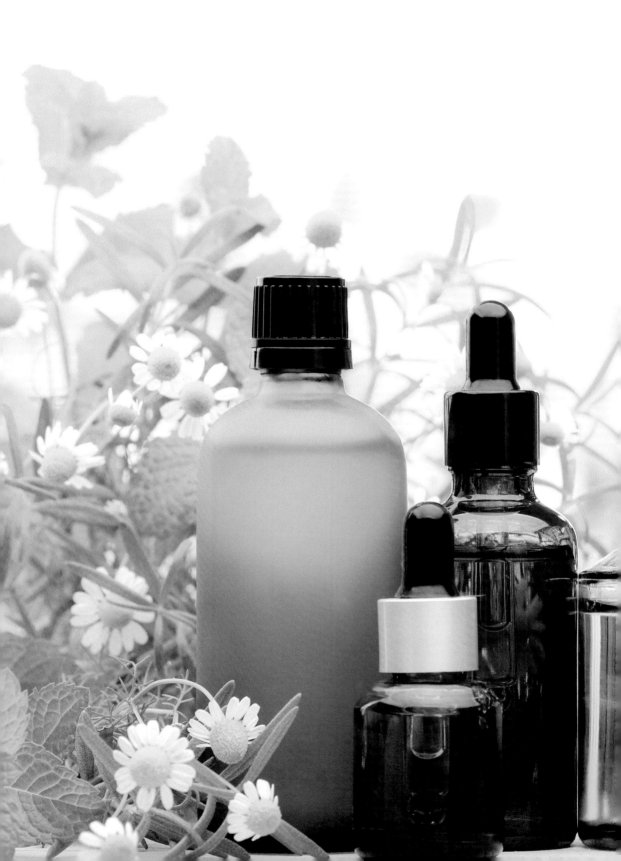

AROMATHERAPY
FORMULAS

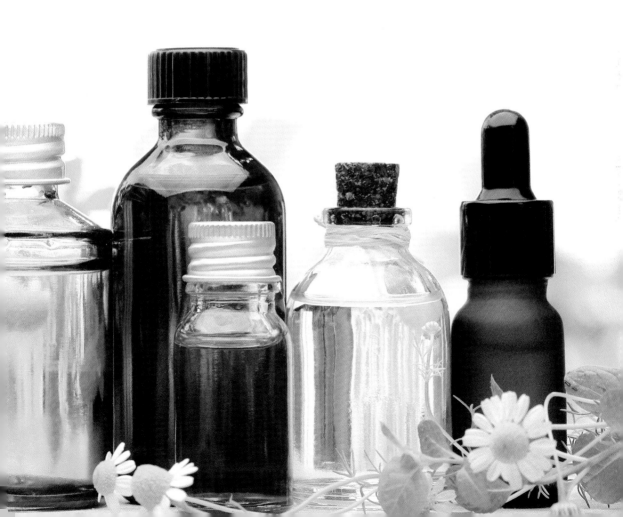

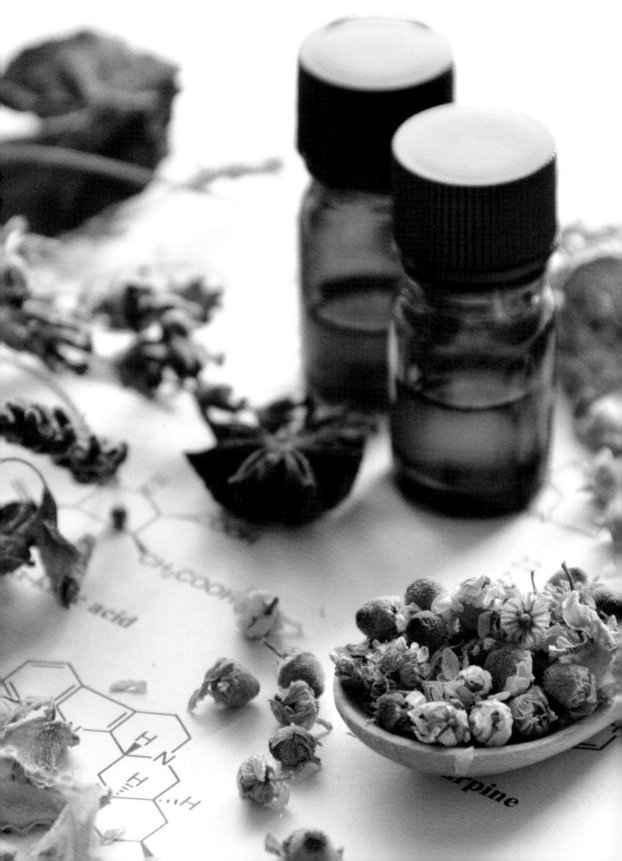

Please review safety guidelines and helpful hints in the Selecting and Using Pure Oils chapter before using the essential oils. Also be sure to follow the blending directions listed in each section for proper use of the formulas.

Air Fresheners

Many of us have experienced elevated moods from smelling the beautiful fragrances of flowers, feeling an ocean breeze, and breathing fresh forest air. Living in big cities, we are deprived of these natural aromas every day. With the use of essential oils, we can recreate the scents we enjoy and bring nature into our homes and offices to enhance our lives.

For All Air Fresheners: Fill a 4-fluid ounce (120 ml) mist spray bottle with purified water, and add the essential oils. Tighten the cap, shake well, and spray the mist into the air. As the mist ages inside the bottle, the scent improves and becomes stronger.

Citrus

lime	50 drops		lime	40 drops
grapefruit	50 drops		lemon	40 drops
orange	10 drops		petitgrain	20 drops
patchouli	10 drops		benzoin	20 drops
pure water	4 fl. oz. (120 ml)		pure water	4 fl. oz. (120 ml)
orange	50 drops		bergamot	50 drops
lemon	35 drops		mandarin	50 drops
grapefruit	20 drops		clove	20 drops
cedarwood	15 drops		pure water	4 fl. oz. (120 ml)
pure water	4 fl. oz. (120 ml)			

Floral

orange	50 drops	geranium	35 drops
rose	25 drops	bois de rose	25 drops
clove	20 drops	rose	25 drops
cinnamon	15 drops	clove	20 drops
jasmine	10 drops	Peru balsam	15 drops
pure water	4 fl. oz. (120 ml)	pure water	4 fl. oz. (120 ml)

rose	75 drops	ylang-ylang	50 drops
orange	25 drops	geranium	25 drops
clove	20 drops	petitgrain	25 drops
pure water	4 fl. oz. (120 ml)	tolu balsam	20 drops
		pure water	4 fl. oz. (120 ml)

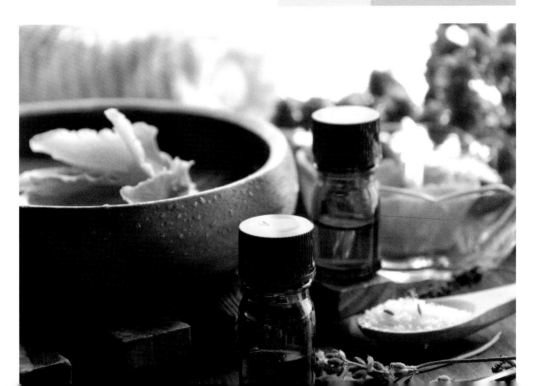

Forest

spruce	50 drops		pine	40 drops
lavender	25 drops		cajeput	40 drops
eucalyptus	25 drops		cypress	20 drops
cedarwood	20 drops		sandalwood	20 drops
pure water	4 fl. oz. (120 ml)		pure water	4 fl. oz. (120 ml)

spruce	40 drops
bois de rose	30 drops
spearmint	30 drops
eucalyptus	20 drops
pure water	4 fl. oz. (120 ml)

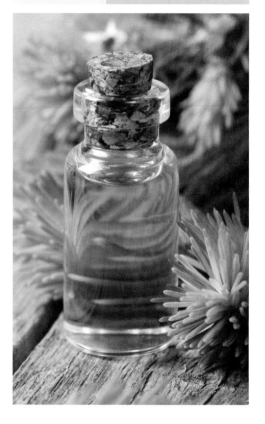

rosemary	30 drops
spruce	30 drops
myrtle	30 drops
lime	15 drops
patchouli	15 drops
pure water	4 fl. oz. (120 ml)

Mint

peppermint	50 drops		*peppermint*	75 drops
spearmint	50 drops		*eucalyptus*	35 drops
Peru balsam	20 drops		*clove*	10 drops
pure water	4 fl. oz. (120 ml)		*pure water*	4 fl. oz. (120 ml)

peppermint	40 drops
caraway	40 drops
petitgrain	20 drops
spearmint	10 drops
patchouli	10 drops
pure water	4 fl. oz. (120 ml)

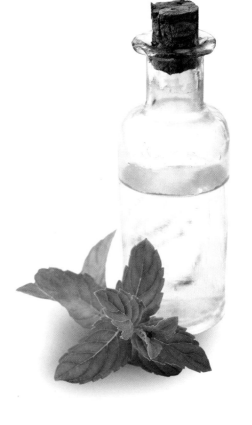

spearmint	40 drops
lavender	30 drops
rosemary	20 drops
benzoin	10 drops
peppermint	10 drops
lime	10 drops
pure water	4 fl. oz. (120 ml)

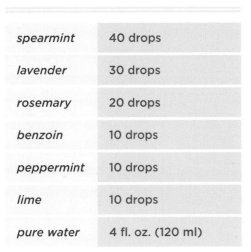

Spice

rosemary	30 drops	peppermint	30 drops
coriander	25 drops	thyme	30 drops
allspice	25 drops	cumin	30 drops
cumin	20 drops	patchouli	20 drops
clove	20 drops	allspice	10 drops
pure water	4 fl. oz. (120 ml)	pure water	4 fl. oz. (120 ml)

marjoram	25 drops	caraway	35 drops
sage	25 drops	anise	20 drops
spearmint	25 drops	cinnamon	20 drops
clove	25 drops	ginger	20 drops
patchouli	20 drops	clove	15 drops
pure water	4 fl. oz. (120 ml)	lime	10 drops
		pure water	4 fl. oz. (120 ml)

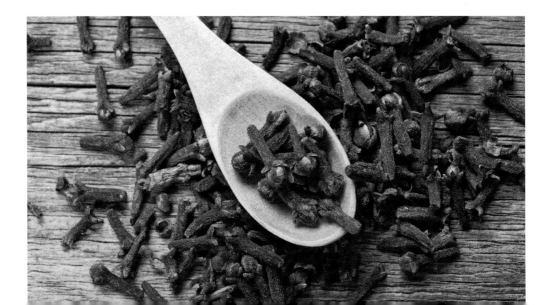

Aroma Lamps

An aroma lamp can be ceramic, marble, glass, or porcelain. It has a small container that is filled with water and is heated by a candle. When essential oils are added to water, aromatic vapor is dispersed into the air. About 15 to 20 drops of essential oil can be used at one time.

Inhale the vapors deeply for best results.

Breathe More Easily

clove	4 drops	spearmint	6 drops
cajeput	4 drops	marjoram	4 drops
myrtle	4 drops	rosemary	4 drops
spruce	4 drops	cubeb	4 drops
lemon	4 drops	lime	2 drops

myrtle	5 drops	lemon	5 drops
lemongrass	5 drops	pine	5 drops
allspice	5 drops	lavender	5 drops
cajeput	5 drops	spearmint	5 drops

pine	6 drops	rosemary	5 drops
lavender	5 drops	cubeb	5 drops
eucalyptus	4 drops	pine	5 drops
cubeb	4 drops	grapefruit	5 drops
lime	1 drop		

Room Disinfectant

pine	6 drops	lemon	5 drops
cinnamon	6 drops	tea tree	5 drops
juniper berries	5 drops	sage	5 drops
clove	3 drops	cajeput	5 drops

eucalyptus	6 drops	clove	6 drops
thyme	6 drops	lime	5 drops
clove	3 drops	allspice	4 drops
lemon	3 drops	cinnamon	4 drops
cinnamon	2 drops	lemon	1 drop

Refreshing

lime	8 drops	pine	8 drops
spearmint	8 drops	spearmint	8 drops
myrtle	4 drops	palmarosa	4 drops

grapefruit	8 drops	peppermint	8 drops
bergamot	4 drops	eucalyptus	8 drops
ginger	4 drops	lemongrass	4 drops
clove	4 drops		

Romance

caraway	5 drops		*clary sage*	5 drops
patchouli	5 drops		*clove*	5 drops
orange	5 drops		*ylang-ylang*	5 drops
benzoin	5 drops		*black pepper*	5 drops

sandalwood	7 drops		*ylang-ylang*	7 drops
ylang-ylang	7 drops		*palmarosa*	7 drops
orange	6 drops		*bergamot*	6 drops

Stress Reduction

melissa	10 drops		*lavender*	10 drops
allspice	10 drops		*mandarin*	10 drops

sandalwood	7 drops		*chamomile*	9 drops
lavender	7 drops		*cinnamon*	6 drops
spruce	6 drops		*fennel*	5 drops

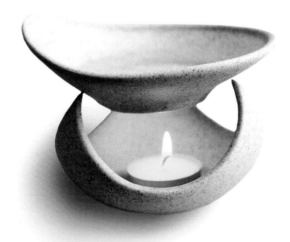

Baby Products

To help protect and soothe your baby's skin from diaper rash, use one of these lavender blends. Apply an ample amount of baby oil on the baby's skin, and store the remaining oil for the next application.

Baby Oil

lavender	5 drops		*lavender*	6 drops
hazelnut	2 tablespoons (30 ml)		*olive*	2 tablespoons (30 ml)

lavender	5 drops		*lavender*	5 drops
flaxseed	2 tablespoons (30 ml)		*sesame*	2 tablespoons (30 ml)

Baby Powder

bois de rose	5 drops
cornstarch	2 tablespoons (30 ml)

lavender	5 drops
cornstarch	2 tablespoons (30 ml)

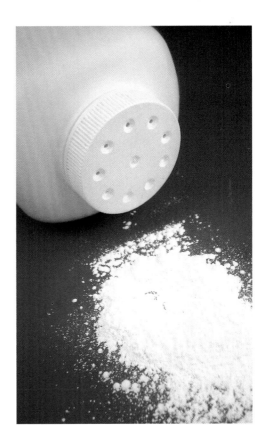

Baths

Besides being necessary for proper hygiene, baths are beneficial to improve one's health. When aromatic oils are added to the bath water, they can help you feel more relaxed and stress-free.

As you prepare your bath, close the window and door to prevent the oil vapors from escaping. Fill the bathtub with warm/hot water. To soften your skin and remove impurities, dissolve 1 cup of Epsom salt in the bath water. Then dilute the essential oils in any of these carrier oils: grapeseed, sweet almond, hazelnut, or sesame. Pour the blend into the water. Swirl the water to disperse the oil evenly. Enter the bath immediately, since essential oils evaporate quickly. Relax and enjoy the bath for at least 30 minutes.

Breathe More Easily

cajeput	5 drops		spruce	5 drops
eucalyptus	5 drops		lavender	5 drops
peppermint	5 drops		cajeput	5 drops
carrier oil	1 teaspoon (5 ml)		carrier oil	1 teaspoon (5 ml)

myrtle	4 drops		myrtle	5 drops
spruce	4 drops		lavender	5 drops
rosemary	4 drops		marjoram	3 drops
grapefruit	3 drops		benzoin	2 drops
carrier oil	1 teaspoon (5 ml)		carrier oil	1 teaspoon (5 ml)

eucalyptus	4 drops		lavender	5 drops
chamomile	4 drops		cajeput	5 drops
anise	3 drops		grapefruit	5 drops
lemon	3 drops		carrier oil	1 teaspoon (5 ml)
petitgrain	1 drop			
carrier oil	1 teaspoon (5 ml)			

Calming

petitgrain	5 drops		*geranium*	5 drops
ylang-ylang	5 drops		*sandalwood*	5 drops
orange	5 drops		*lemon*	5 drops
carrier oil	1 teaspoon (5 ml)		*carrier oil*	1 teaspoon (5 ml)

cypress	5 drops		*chamomile*	5 drops
marjoram	3 drops		*geranium*	5 drops
melissa	3 drops		*clary sage*	2 drops
lemon	3 drops		*lemon*	2 drops
geranium	1 drop		*Peru balsam*	1 drop
carrier oil	1 teaspoon (5 ml)		*carrier oil*	1 teaspoon (5 ml)

petitgrain	5 drops		*allspice*	5 drops
lavender	5 drops		*chamomile*	5 drops
fennel	3 drops		*mandarin*	5 drops
orange	2 drops		*carrier oil*	1 teaspoon (5 ml)
carrier oil	1 teaspoon (5 ml)			

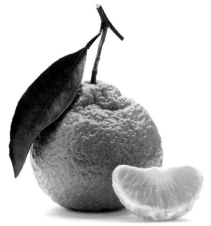

Mood Elevating

bois de rose	5 drops		geranium	5 drops
palmarosa	5 drops		bergamot	4 drops
grapefruit	3 drops		allspice	3 drops
petitgrain	2 drops		orange	3 drops
carrier oil	1 teaspoon (5 ml)		carrier oil	1 teaspoon (5 ml)

ylang-ylang	5 drops		bergamot	5 drops
sandalwood	5 drops		rosemary	5 drops
grapefruit	5 drops		benzoin	5 drops
carrier oil	1 teaspoon (5 ml)		carrier oil	1 teaspoon (5 ml)

clary sage	3 drops		patchouli	4 drops
bois de rose	3 drops		bergamot	3 drops
lime	3 drops		clary sage	3 drops
patchouli	3 drops		geranium	3 drops
geranium	3 drops		palmarosa	2 drops
carrier oil	1 teaspoon (5 ml)		carrier oil	1 teaspoon (5 ml)

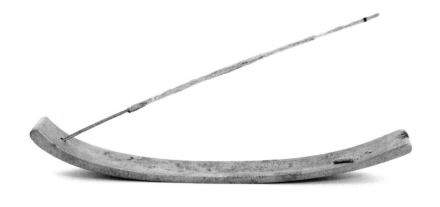

Muscle Relaxers

cedarwood	4 drops		cypress	5 drops
chamomile	4 drops		sandalwood	5 drops
lavender	4 drops		nutmeg	3 drops
lemongrass	3 drops		lavender	2 drops
carrier oil	1 teaspoon (5 ml)		carrier oil	1 teaspoon (5 ml)

cypress	5 drops		allspice	5 drops
marjoram	3 drops		petitgrain	5 drops
lavender	3 drops		ylang-ylang	5 drops
sweet basil	2 drops		carrier oil	1 teaspoon (5 ml)
cedarwood	2 drops			
carrier oil	1 teaspoon (5 ml)			

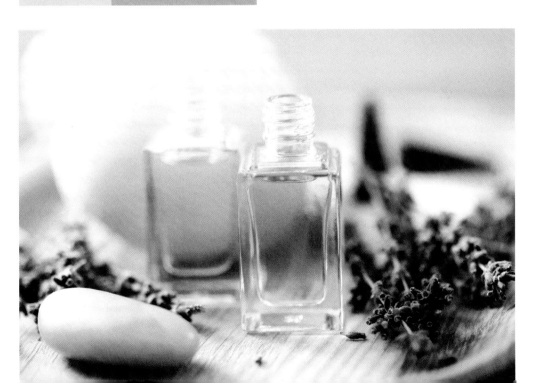

Premenstrual Syndrome

grapefruit	4 drops		bergamot	4 drops
clary sage	4 drops		fennel	4 drops
ylang-ylang	4 drops		bois de rose	4 drops
geranium	3 drops		melissa	3 drops
carrier oil	1 teaspoon (5 ml)		carrier oil	1 teaspoon (5 ml)

bergamot	5 drops
geranium	5 drops
palmarosa	5 drops
carrier oil	1 teaspoon (5 ml)

allspice	5 drops
lemon	4 drops
chamomile	3 drops
geranium	3 drops
carrier oil	1 teaspoon (5 ml)

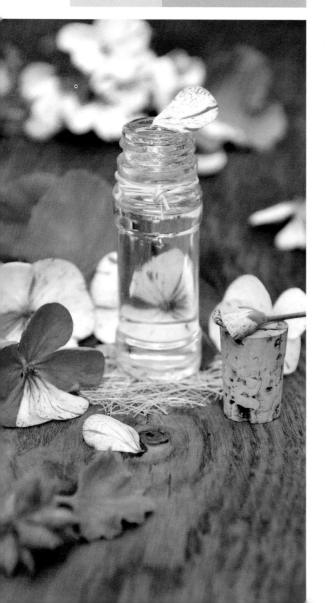

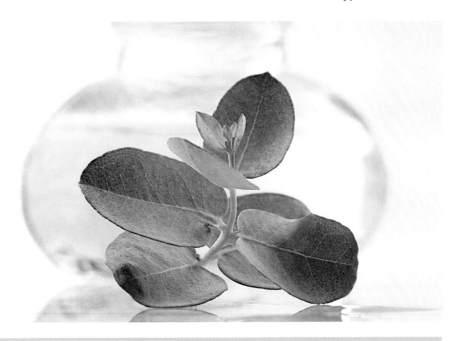

Refreshing

bergamot	4 drops		lavender	5 drops
eucalyptus	4 drops		peppermint	4 drops
melissa	4 drops		grapefruit	3 drops
peppermint	3 drops		lemongrass	3 drops
carrier oil	1 teaspoon (5 ml)		carrier oil	1 teaspoon (5 ml)

lavender	5 drops		spruce	4 drops
bergamot	3 drops		geranium	4 drops
lime	3 drops		spearmint	4 drops
cypress	2 drops		juniper berries	2 drops
cajeput	2 drops		lemon	2 drops
carrier oil	1 teaspoon (5 ml)		carrier oil	1 teaspoon (5 ml)

Stress Relievers

allspice	5 drops	sandalwood	5 drops
rosemary	4 drops	fennel	3 drops
fennel	2 drops	melissa	3 drops
cypress	2 drops	sweet basil	2 drops
mandarin	2 drops	lavender	2 drops
carrier oil	1 teaspoon (5 ml)	carrier oil	1 teaspoon (5 ml)

marjoram	4 drops
cedarwood	4 drops
melissa	3 drops
grapefruit	2 drops
orange	2 drops
carrier oil	1 teaspoon (5 ml)

lavender	3 drops
chamomile	3 drops
melissa	3 drops
cedarwood	3 drops
mandarin	3 drops
carrier oil	1 teaspoon (5 ml)

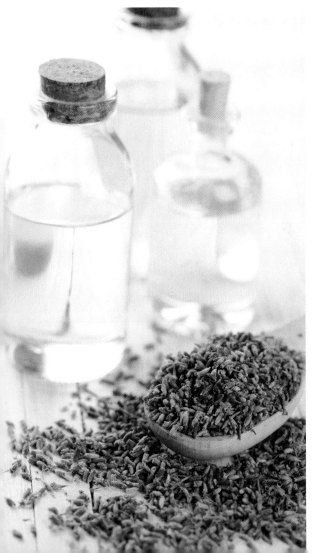

Body Powder

Measure the amount of cornstarch and pour into a wide-mouthed glass jar or a spice powder container; then add the essential oils. Tighten the cap and let the body powder sit for a day. Shake well before using.

Citrus Scent

mandarin	12 drops		*bergamot*	15 drops
lemon	12 drops		*grapefruit*	10 drops
patchouli	6 drops		*sandalwood*	5 drops
cornstarch	2 tablespoons (30 ml)		cornstarch	2 tablespoons (30 ml)

grapefruit	15 drops		*lemon*	20 drops
lime	10 drops		*lavender*	5 drops
allspice	5 drops		*allspice*	5 drops
cornstarch	2 tablespoons (30 ml)		cornstarch	2 tablespoons (30 ml)

lime	10 drops		*petitgrain*	15 drops
orange	10 drops		*neroli*	15 drops
clove	5 drops		cornstarch	2 tablespoons (30 ml)
petitgrain	5 drops			
cornstarch	2 tablespoons (30 ml)			

Floral Scent

bois de rose	10 drops		jasmine	10 drops
lavender	10 drops		bois de rose	10 drops
mandarin	5 drops		rose	5 drops
ylang-ylang	5 drops		clove	5 drops
cornstarch	2 tablespoons (30 ml)		cornstarch	2 tablespoons (30 ml)

rose	20 drops		ylang-ylang	20 drops
orange	10 drops		geranium	10 drops
cornstarch	2 tablespoons (30 ml)		cornstarch	2 tablespoons (30 ml)

geranium	10 drops		ylang-ylang	10 drops
bergamot	10 drops		melissa	5 drops
ylang-ylang	10 drops		clove	5 drops
cornstarch	2 tablespoons (30 ml)		nutmeg	5 drops
			orange	5 drops
			cornstarch	2 tablespoons (30 ml)

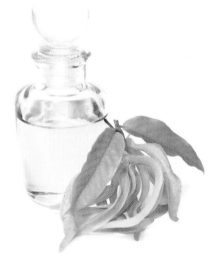

Forest Scent

spruce	10 drops		sandalwood	10 drops
cedarwood	10 drops		chamomile	10 drops
juniper berries	5 drops		rosemary	5 drops
cajeput	5 drops		lemon	5 drops
cornstarch	2 tablespoons (30 ml)		cornstarch	2 tablespoons (30 ml)

pine	15 drops		cypress	10 drops
spruce	10 drops		eucalyptus	10 drops
spearmint	5 drops		sandalwood	10 drops
cornstarch	2 tablespoons (30 ml)		cornstarch	2 tablespoons (30 ml)

eucalyptus	10 drops		sage	10 drops
juniper berries	10 drops		patchouli	5 drops
myrtle	5 drops		cedarwood	5 drops
lemon	5 drops		spruce	5 drops
cornstarch	2 tablespoons (30 ml)		lavender	5 drops
			cornstarch	2 tablespoons (30 ml)

Minty Scent

peppermint	10 drops		spearmint	15 drops
spruce	10 drops		lemon	5 drops
clove	5 drops		patchouli	5 drops
spearmint	5 drops		lavender	5 drops
cornstarch	2 tablespoons (30 ml)		cornstarch	2 tablespoons (30 ml)

peppermint	15 drops		spearmint	15 drops
caraway	10 drops		lavender	10 drops
lavender	5 drops		sweet bay	5 drops
cornstarch	2 tablespoons (30 ml)		cornstarch	2 tablespoons (30 ml)

Spicy Scent

allspice	15 drops
caraway	10 drops
lavender	5 drops
cornstarch	2 tablespoons (30 ml)

caraway	10 drops
clove	10 drops
rosemary	10 drops
cornstarch	2 tablespoons (30 ml)

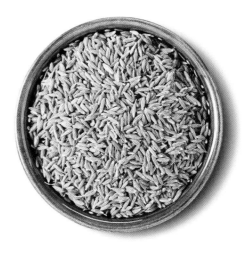

Breath Fresheners

Mix all ingredients in a mist sprayer, shake well before using, then mist once or twice directly into the mouth.

peppermint	10 drops		cinnamon	10 drops
spearmint	10 drops		orange	10 drops
pure water	4 fl. oz (120 ml)		pure water	4 fl. oz (120 ml)
honey	½ teaspoon (2.5 ml)		honey	½ teaspoon (2.5 ml)

peppermint	10 drops		pine	10 drops
lavender	5 drops		anise	5 drops
clove	5 drops		lavender	5 drops
pure water	4 fl. oz (120 ml)		pure water	4 fl. oz (120 ml)
honey	½ teaspoon (2.5 ml)		honey	½ teaspoon (2.5 ml)

spearmint	10 drops		lemon	10 drops
lime	10 drops		lavender	10 drops
pure water	4 fl. oz (120 ml)		pure water	4 fl. oz (120 ml)
honey	½ teaspoon (2.5 ml)		honey	½ teaspoon (2.5 ml)

allspice	10 drops		chamomile	10 drops
lemon	5 drops		allspice	5 drops
anise	5 drops		pine	5 drops
pure water	4 fl. oz (120 ml)		pure water	4 fl. oz (120 ml)
honey	½ teaspoon (2.5 ml)		honey	½ teaspoon (2.5 ml)

Candles

You can create a delightful atmosphere by burning a candle scented with essential oils. Place several drops of the oil on the wax before lighting the candle. Avoid dropping the oil into the flame or on the wick. For thick candles, heat a metal ice pick and pierce a hole through the wax and add essential oils. Select your favorite oil(s) from one of the scent categories.

Citrus Scent	
	grapefruit
	lemon
	lemongrass
	lime
	melissa
	neroli
	orange

Minty Scent	
	peppermint
	spearmint

Spicy Scent	
	allspice
	caraway
	clove
	sage

Floral Scent	
	benzoin
	jasmine
	rose
	tolu balsam
	ylang-ylang

Forest Scent	
	eucalyptus
	myrtle
	pine
	rosemary
	spruce

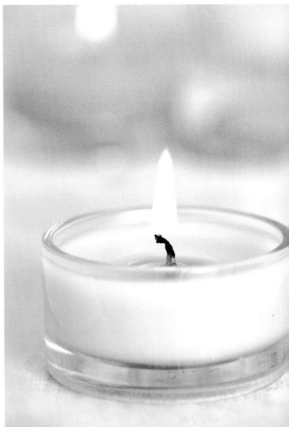

Carpet Fresheners

Mix all ingredients in a wide-mouthed glass jar and tighten the cap. Set aside for 24 hours to allow the aromas to permeate the powder. Sprinkle over carpeting, leave for 10 to 15 minutes, and vacuum.

lavender	60 drops		rosemary	60 drops
cinnamon	20 drops		spruce	30 drops
orange	20 drops		orange	10 drops
bicarbonate of soda	½ cup (120 ml)		bicarbonate of soda	½ cup (120 ml)
clove	60 drops		lime	50 drops
peppermint	20 drops		orange	30 drops
dill	20 drops		patchouli	20 drops
bicarbonate of soda	½ cup (120 ml)		bicarbonate of soda	½ cup (120 ml)
eucalyptus	30 drops		anise	40 drops
cinnamon	30 drops		clove	40 drops
lemongrass	30 drops		patchouli	20 drops
clove	10 drops		bicarbonate of soda	½ cup (120 ml)
bicarbonate of soda	½ cup (120 ml)			

Chapped Lips (Lip Balm)

These formulas should be very helpful to moisturize chapped lips.

Heat a small pot of water on a low temperature, place the shea butter into a small wide-mouthed glass jar, and place the jar into the pot of water. When the shea butter is melted, add the carrier oil (sesame oil), mix well, and remove from the heat. As the mixture cools, add the essential oils and stir well. Refrigerate the jar. The crème can take over an hour to thicken. When it completely cools, remove from the refrigerator, stir the lip balm, and let sit at room temperature for a few hours. Check the thickness. Once the lip balm is at room temperature, and if you prefer to make it thicker, melt additional shea butter and add to the crème. If you'd like to make it thinner, add more carrier oil. Label the jar. Store in a dark, cool place.

To use: Apply aloe vera gel or juice on the lips, then the lip balm creme, several times daily as needed.

bois de rose	15 drops
lavender	5 drops
frankincense	5 drops
shea butter	3 tablespoons (45 ml)
sesame	1 tablespoon (15 ml)

chamomile	10 drops
elemi	10 drops
ylang-ylang	5 drops
shea butter	3 tablespoons (45 ml)
sesame	1 tablespoon (15 ml)

palmarosa	15 drops
ylang-ylang	5 drops
patchouli	5 drops
shea butter	3 tablespoons (45 ml)
sesame	1 tablespoon (15 ml)

palmarosa	15 drops
ylang-ylang	5 drops
bois de rose	5 drops
shea butter	3 tablespoons (45 ml)
sesame	1 tablespoon (15 ml)

bois de rose	20 drops
myrrh	5 drops
shea butter	3 tablespoons (45 ml)
sesame	1 tablespoon (15 ml)

sandalwood	15 drops
elemi	10 drops
shea butter	3 tablespoons (45 ml)
sesame	1 tablespoon (15 ml)

palmarosa	15 drops
chamomile	10 drops
shea butter	3 tablespoons (45 ml)
sesame	1 tablespoon (15 ml)

sandalwood	10 drops
rose	5 drops
myrrh	5 drops
bois de rose	5 drops
shea butter	3 tablespoons (45 ml)
sesame	1 tablespoon (15 ml)

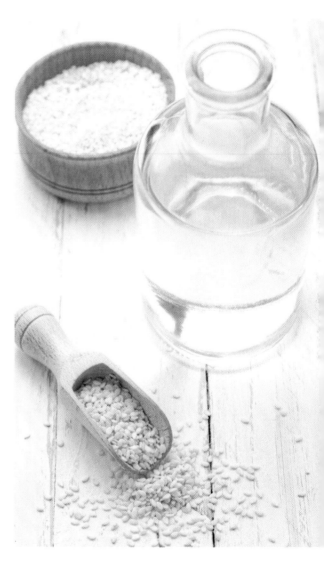

Closet and Drawer Scents

Put 10 drops of your favorite essential oil on a cotton ball and place it inside a plastic bag. Leave the bag open and place it in a closet or dresser drawer to scent your clothing. When the scent wears off, repeat again with additional drops.

Deodorants

Foot Deodorizer

Some people experience unpleasant odors from their feet. These formulas will keep the feet smelling fresh. Select one of the formulas, and use the entire blend on each foot. Finish by dabbing on cornstarch to dry any remaining oil on the skin. Apply daily if needed.

sesame	20 drops		*sesame*	20 drops
tolu balsam	3 drops		*tolu balsam*	3 drops
cypress	2 drops		*bergamot*	3 drops
lavender	2 drops			

Underarm Deodorant Roll-On

Choose one of these formulas. Place the essential oils into a glass roll-on bottle and label the bottle.
To use: Apply five drops of aloe vera gel or juice to each underarm, then roll on the deodorant.
To dry any remaining oil from the skin, rub on a small amount of cornstarch or arrowroot powder. The roll-on formula should last for many applications.

Please note: After a woman shaves her underarms, it is advisable to wait at least 15 minutes before applying the deodorant to avoid any possible burning sensation.

spikenard	40 drops		*champaca flower*	45 drops
bois de rose	25 drops		*spikenard*	40 drops
guaiacwood	25 drops		*vanilla CO$_2$*	25 drops
sage	20 drops			

spikenard	40 drops
guaiacwood	40 drops
bois de rose	30 drops

bois de rose	45 drops
guaiacwood	40 drops
vanilla CO$_2$	15 drops

champaca flower	55 drops
guaiacwood	40 drops
sage	15 drops

spikenard	50 drops
vanilla CO$_2$	50 drops
sage	10 drops

champaca flower	65 drops
spikenard	45 drops

bois de rose	80 drops
vanilla CO$_2$	30 drops

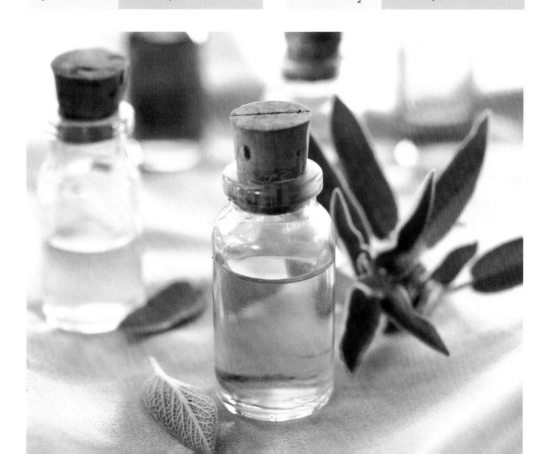

Diffusers

Diffusers have become popular during the last few years. These devices disperse a fine mist of the microparticles of essential oils which purifies and revitalizes the indoor atmosphere. Electric diffusers are especially wonderful for large rooms and office buildings, since the mist is continuously diffused into the air.

Thick or resinous oils will cause damage to the nebulizer; therefore, choose from the following oils.

Breathe More Easily	
cajeput	peppermint
clove	pine
eucalyptus	spearmint
juniper berries	spruce
lavender	tea tree
myrtle	

Disinfectant	
allspice	lavender
bergamot	pine
cajeput	rosemary
cinnamon	sage
clove	tea tree
eucalyptus	thyme

Energizing	
eucalyptus	peppermint
lemon	pine
lime	spearmint

Stress-Free	
allspice	lemon
bois de rose	mandarin
chamomile	melissa
geranium	neroli
grapefruit	orange
lavender	petitgrain

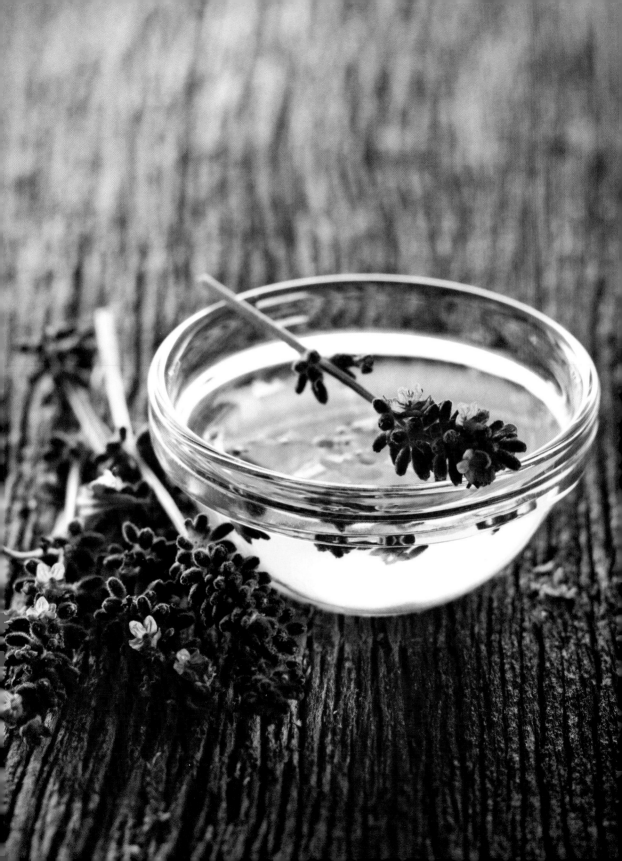

Foot Baths

Select a carrier oil—grapeseed, sweet almond, hazelnut, or sesame—to dilute the essential oils. Then fill the basin with warm water, and add one of the formulas below. Swirl the water to disperse the blended oils and relax for at least 15 minutes.

Rejuvenating

cubeb	3 drops		cypress	4 drops
geranium	3 drops		lemon	4 drops
thyme	3 drops		palmarosa	3 drops
allspice	3 drops		cinnamon	2 drops
pine	3 drops		eucalyptus	2 drops
carrier oil	1 teaspoon (5 ml)		carrier oil	1 teaspoon (5 ml)

sandalwood	3 drops		thyme	3 drops
black pepper	3 drops		peppermint	3 drops
spruce	3 drops		lemongrass	3 drops
geranium	3 drops		geranium	3 drops
grapefruit	3 drops		lavender	3 drops
carrier oil	1 teaspoon (5 ml)		carrier oil	1 teaspoon (5 ml)

lemon	5 drops		ginger	4 drops
spearmint	4 drops		lime	4 drops
black pepper	3 drops		geranium	4 drops
pine	3 drops		spearmint	3 drops
carrier oil	1 teaspoon (5 ml)		carrier oil	1 teaspoon (5 ml)

myrtle	4 drops
spearmint	4 drops
grapefruit	4 drops
cajeput	3 drops
carrier oil	1 teaspoon (5 ml)

eucalyptus	4 drops
pine	4 drops
peppermint	4 drops
geranium	3 drops
carrier oil	1 teaspoon (5 ml)

Relaxing

mandarin	4 drops
lavender	4 drops
anise	2 drops
sweet basil	2 drops
petitgrain	2 drops
lemon	1 drop
carrier oil	1 teaspoon (5 ml)

geranium	4 drops
cedarwood	3 drops
marjoram	3 drops
clary sage	2 drops
benzoin	2 drops
celery	1 drop
carrier oil	1 teaspoon (5 ml)

petitgrain	5 drops
lemon	4 drops
fennel	3 drops
cinnamon	2 drops
melissa	1 drop
carrier oil	1 teaspoon (5 ml)

dill	3 drops
grapefruit	3 drops
allspice	3 drops
spruce	3 drops
anise	3 drops
carrier oil	1 teaspoon (5 ml)

Relaxing *(continued)*

marjoram	4 drops		myrrh	4 drops
petitgrain	4 drops		chamomile	4 drops
ylang-ylang	4 drops		orange	4 drops
Peru balsam	3 drops		lemon	3 drops
carrier oil	1 teaspoon (5 ml)		carrier oil	1 teaspoon (5 ml)

lemongrass	3 drops		frankincense	4 drops
melissa	3 drops		neroli	4 drops
allspice	3 drops		anise	4 drops
geranium	3 drops		lemon	3 drops
nutmeg	3 drops		carrier oil	1 teaspoon (5 ml)
carrier oil	1 teaspoon (5 ml)			

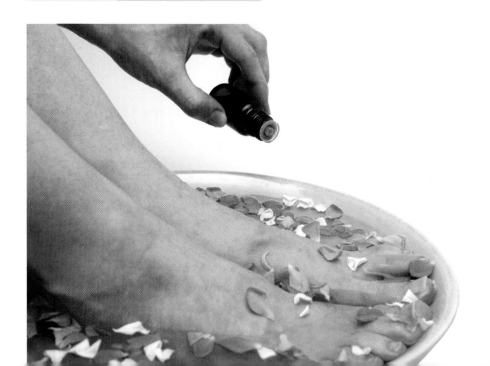

Foot Powder

Measure the amount of cornstarch, and pour it into a wide-mouthed glass jar or a spice powder container. Then add the essential oils. Tighten the cap, and let the foot powder sit for a day. Shake before using. Before applying the powder, rub in well at least 5 drops of grapeseed oil with 3 drops of tolu balsam on the bottom of each foot. Use a small amount of powder at one time.

peppermint	15 drops		*spearmint*	15 drops
lemon	10 drops		*mandarin*	10 drops
cinnamon	5 drops		*geranium*	5 drops
cornstarch	2 tablespoons (30 ml)		*cornstarch*	2 tablespoons (30 ml)

chamomile	20 drops		*ylang-ylang*	10 drops
clove	5 drops		*ginger*	10 drops
sweet bay	5 drops		*lemon*	10 drops
cornstarch	2 tablespoons (30 ml)		*cornstarch*	2 tablespoons (30 ml)

grapefruit	10 drops		*cypress*	10 drops
spruce	10 drops		*eucalyptus*	10 drops
patchouli	5 drops		*clove*	5 drops
lemongrass	5 drops		*orange*	5 drops
cornstarch	2 tablespoons (30 ml)		*cornstarch*	2 tablespoons (30 ml)

Furniture Polish

Use this polish on your furniture for a beautiful shine. Combine ingredients and gently polish. Use a small amount of powder at one time.

ylang-ylang	10 drops
jojoba	1 fluid ounce (30 ml)

Gardening

E ssential oils can strengthen plants and repel insects at the same time.

Fill a container with water; then add the essential oils. Mix well to disperse the oil droplets in the water. Water plants well prior to using one of these solutions. Use small amounts around the drip line of the plant.

sage	10 drops	thyme	10 drops
clove	5 drops	lavender	5 drops
water	1 gallon (3.8 L)	water	1 gallon (3.8 L)

cinnamon	8 drops	clove	10 drops
peppermint	7 drops	sweet bay	5 drops
water	1 gallon (3.8 L)	water	1 gallon (3.8 L)

If your plants or bushes are *already* infested with insects, use one of the strong solutions below. Fill the mist spray bottle with water, then add the essential oils. Tighten the cap, shake well, and mist the infested plant. Use as minimal an amount as possible. Several applications, a few days apart, may be necessary. These mist sprays can be used on outdoor or indoor plants:

sage	45 drops	lavender	50 drops
thyme	45 drops	fennel	40 drops
water	4 fl. oz. (120 ml)	water	4 fl. oz. (120 ml)

peppermint	45 drops	cinnamon	50 drops
sweet bay	45 drops	patchouli	40 drops
water	4 fl. oz. (120 ml)	water	4 fl. oz. (120 ml)

clove	45 drops	coriander	45 drops
caraway	45 drops	lavender	45 drops
water	4 fl. oz. (120 ml)	water	4 fl. oz. (120 ml)

Hair Care

The condition of your hair is very important to the way you look. Regardless of the style, your hair should be thick, shiny, and soft. These formulas will help promote a natural shine in your hair.

Massage approximately 1 teaspoon into your hair and scalp at one time. It's best to leave on for several hours to allow the oils to penetrate. If you use the formula before bedtime, wrap a towel around your head, and leave on overnight. In the morning, wash your hair twice with a natural shampoo (available in health food stores) and warm water. Use the formula three times a week, until you achieve desired results. It is best to discontinue use of commercial shampoos and harsh chemicals on the hair and scalp to maintain beautiful, shiny hair.

Normal Hair

cedarwood	8 drops	thyme	8 drops
rosemary	8 drops	sage	6 drops
sweet bay	8 drops	chamomile	6 drops
geranium	3 drops	lavender	5 drops
jojoba	2 tablespoons (30 ml)	jojoba	2 tablespoons (30 ml)

Dry Hair

sandalwood	10 drops	ginger	10 drops
bois de rose	10 drops	bois de rose	10 drops
palmarosa	5 drops	lavender	5 drops
jojoba	2 tablespoons (30 ml)	sesame	2 tablespoons (30 ml)

Oily Hair

ylang-ylang	9 drops	petitgrain	8 drops
lime	9 drops	lemon	8 drops
rosemary	8 drops	lavender	8 drops
grapeseed	2 tablespoons (30 ml)	hazelnut	2 tablespoons (30 ml)

Hand Baths

Those people who experience tired and aching hands after a day's work may find relief in one of these hand baths. Select a carrier oil—grapeseed, sweet almond, hazelnut, or sesame—to dilute the essential oils. Add the blend of oils to a basin of warm water and soak your hands for 20 to 30 minutes.

Soothe Aching Muscles

spearmint	5 drops		melissa	5 drops
palmarosa	5 drops		lavender	5 drops
geranium	5 drops		allspice	5 drops
carrier oil	1 teaspoon (5 ml)		carrier oil	1 teaspoon (5 ml)

peppermint	4 drops		cypress	5 drops
thyme	4 drops		cinnamon	4 drops
lavender	4 drops		cajeput	4 drops
marjoram	3 drops		lemon	2 drops
carrier oil	1 teaspoon (5 ml)		carrier oil	1 teaspoon (5 ml)

sweet bay	4 drops		geranium	5 drops
ginger	4 drops		ylang-ylang	4 drops
ylang-ylang	4 drops		spearmint	4 drops
lavender	3 drops		lavender	2 drops
carrier oil	1 teaspoon (5 ml)		carrier oil	1 teaspoon (5 ml)

Insect Bites

These formulas help to soothe the area of the insect bite and relieve discomfort. Apply the formula to the bite every few hours.

aloe vera gel	1 teaspoon (5 ml)
geranium	5 drops

aloe vera gel	1 teaspoon (5 ml)
chamomile	5 drops

sesame	1 teaspoon (5 ml)
juniper berries	2 drops
sweet basil	2 drops
lime	1 drop

borage	1 teaspoon (5 ml)
juniper berries	2 drops
tea tree	2 drops
lemon	1 drop

flaxseed	1 teaspoon (5 ml)
sweet basil	2 drops
lemon	2 drops
marjoram	1 drop

aloe vera gel	1 teaspoon (5 ml)
lavender	5 drops

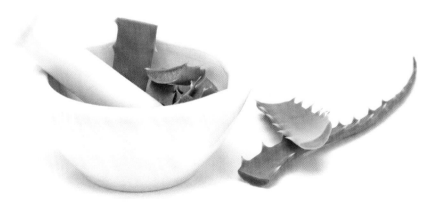

Insect Repellents

To deter insects, spray the mist on the exposed areas of the body before going outdoors. Rub jojoba oil into the skin prior to spraying the formula. Spray a minimal amount. Avoid misting on the face; instead, apply this face oil: patchouli—4 drops, cajeput—4 drops, basil (sweet)—2 drops blended in 2 teaspoons of carrier oil.

jojoba	100 drops
lavender	100 drops
eucalyptus	50 drops
lemongrass	50 drops
patchouli	50 drops
cajeput	50 drops
vodka	2 fl. oz. (60 ml)

jojoba	100 drops
geranium	100 drops
cedarwood	50 drops
sweet bay	50 drops
lime	50 drops
pine	50 drops
vodka	2 fl. oz. (60 ml)

jojoba	100 drops
cajeput	100 drops
lavender	100 drops
patchouli	100 drops
vodka	2 fl. oz. (60 ml)

jojoba	100 drops
cedarwood	75 drops
patchouli	75 drops
lime	50 drops
lavender	50 drops
geranium	50 drops
vodka	2 fl. oz. (60 ml)

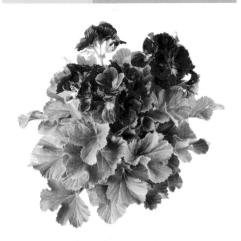

Hot Tub Oils

Add 5 drops of essential oil per person. If only one person will be in the Jacuzzi, increase the amount of oil to 10 drops. Select your favorite oil or choose one of these.

chamomile	*eucalyptus*	*geranium*
lavender	*myrtle*	*pine*
spearmint	*spruce*	*tea tree*

Lactation

Massage the entire blend into the upper chest. Then rub cornstarch over the same area to absorb any oily residue, since this residue could irritate a baby's tender skin, while nursing.

To Increase Lactation	
lemongrass	5 drops
sesame	1 teaspoon (5 ml)

To Decrease Lactation	
peppermint	5 drops
grapeseed	1 teaspoon (5 ml)
sage	5 drops
grapeseed	1 teaspoon (5 ml)

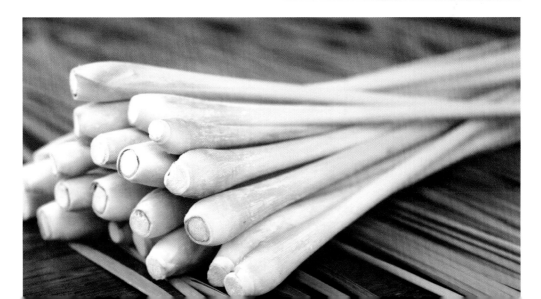

Laundry Scents

Put 10 drops of essential oil on a cotton cloth, and place the cloth in the dryer together with the clothes to be scented. Choose any one of these oils.

clove	lime	spearmint
geranium	peppermint	spruce
lavender		

Lice Removers

Lice are common parasites that infest the hair. These formulas help kill lice and nourish the hair and scalp, as well.

Massage the entire formula vigorously into the hair and scalp before bedtime. Wrap a towel around the head, and leave it on overnight. Repeat nightly until the lice are gone.

thyme	5 drops
rosemary	5 drops
lavender	5 drops
jojoba	1 tablespoon (15 ml)

ginger	5 drops
rosemary	5 drops
cajeput	5 drops
walnut	1 tablespoon (15 ml)

peppermint	5 drops
ginger	5 drops
lavender	5 drops
walnut	1 tablespoon (15 ml)

geranium	8 drops
rosemary	7 drops
jojoba	1 tablespoon (15 ml)

Light Bulb Rings

The brass ring rests on top of the light bulb and diffuses the desired aroma when the bulb is hot. Choose an oil from one of the scent categories below.

Place five drops of essential oil in the ring before turning on the light. Avoid adding oil when the bulb is hot, since it may shatter. Use only light bulbs that are 60 watts or lower.

Citrus Scent	grapefruit
	lemon
	lemongrass
	lime
	melissa
	neroli
	orange

| Minty Scent | peppermint |
| | spearmint |

Spicy Scent	allspice
	caraway
	clove
	sage

Floral Scent	benzoin
	jasmine
	rose
	tolu balsam
	ylang-ylang

Forest Scent	eucalyptus
	myrtle
	pine
	rosemary
	spruce

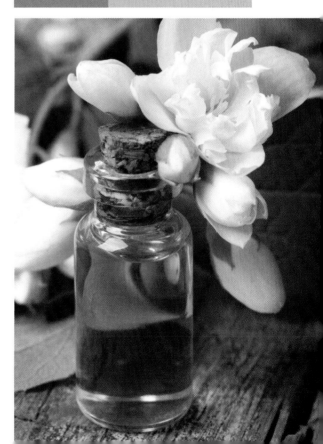

Massage Oils

When applying essential oils on the skin, a carrier oil should always be added to the blend. The importance of using a carrier oil is to dilute the essential oils in order to protect the skin from becoming irritated. Combine the carrier oil with the essential oils, in a small glass bottle. Before using, gently shake the bottle to mix the oils together. Then pour a portion of the oil into one palm, rub both palms together to distribute the oil evenly, and apply to the person's skin. Gradually massage the blend into the specific areas of the body. If the person has dry or sensitive skin, additional carrier oil may be necessary. For best results, all massage formulas should be massaged for at least 30 minutes, until all the oil is fully absorbed by the skin. To remove any oil residue after the treatment, rub cornstarch on the area.

If a specific carrier oil is indicated in the massage formula, be sure to use that carrier. If a carrier oil is not specified, choose one from the following list.

sweet almond	*flaxseed*	*jojoba*	*olive*
avocado	*grapeseed*	*kukui nut*	*sesame*
borage*	*hazelnut*	*macadamia nut*	*walnut*

*Dilute with another carrier oil.

Ache and Pain Relievers

Massage the formula into the specific area(s).

rosemary	5 drops
caraway	5 drops
lavender	5 drops
carrier oil	1 tablespoon (15 ml)

cardamom	5 drops
eucalyptus	5 drops
pine	5 drops
carrier oil	1 tablespoon (15 ml)

ginger	5 drops
sweet bay	5 drops
marjoram	5 drops
carrier oil	1 tablespoon (15 ml)

peppermint	5 drops
allspice	5 drops
marjoram	5 drops
carrier oil	1 tablespoon (15 ml)

Calming

Massage the blend into the shoulders, back of the neck, and down the back.

petitgrain	6 drops	ylang-ylang	5 drops
orange	5 drops	orange	5 drops
neroli	4 drops	petitgrain	5 drops
carrier oil	1 tablespoon (15 ml)	carrier oil	1 tablespoon (15 ml)

bois de rose	5 drops	myrrh	4 drops
anise	4 drops	mandarin	4 drops
cajeput	4 drops	spruce	4 drops
sweet basil	2 drops	neroli	3 drops
carrier oil	1 tablespoon (15 ml)	carrier oil	1 tablespoon (15 ml)

petitgrain	5 drops	chamomile	5 drops
cedarwood	5 drops	bergamot	5 drops
chamomile	5 drops	lavender	5 drops
carrier oil	1 tablespoon (15 ml)	carrier oil	1 tablespoon (15 ml)

cedarwood	5 drops	melissa	5 drops
lemon	5 drops	allspice	5 drops
mandarin	5 drops	elemi	5 drops
carrier oil	1 tablespoon (15 ml)	carrier oil	1 tablespoon (15 ml)

Calming *(continued)*

sandalwood	5 drops		*cedarwood*	5 drops
bois de rose	4 drops		*clary sage*	4 drops
lavender	4 drops		*palmarosa*	4 drops
lemongrass	2 drops		*lemon*	2 drops
carrier oil	1 tablespoon (15 ml)		*carrier oil*	1 tablespoon (15 ml)

Cellulite Reduction

Many people have cellulite. With the use of these cellulite-reducing blends and a wholesome diet, reducing weight and inches is feasible. Massage the formula into the cellulite area(s). Work deeply into the tissues to help smooth bumpy and dimpled skin.

celery	5 drops		*rosemary*	5 drops
grapefruit	5 drops		*ginger*	5 drops
cinnamon	5 drops		*coriander*	5 drops
benzoin	5 drops		*lemon*	5 drops
carrier oil	4 teaspoons (20 ml)		*carrier oil*	4 teaspoons (20 ml)

geranium	5 drops		*grapefruit*	5 drops
celery	5 drops		*pine*	5 drops
lime	5 drops		*cinnamon*	5 drops
benzoin	3 drops		*fennel*	3 drops
black pepper	2 drops		*cypress*	2 drops
carrier oil	4 teaspoons (20 ml)		*carrier oil*	4 teaspoons (20 ml)

coriander	5 drops
lavender	5 drops
thyme	5 drops
grapefruit	5 drops
carrier oil	4 teaspoons (20 ml)

cypress	5 drops
rosemary	5 drops
benzoin	5 drops
sweet basil	4 drops
carrier oil	4 teaspoons (20 ml)

rosemary	4 drops
celery	4 drops
cypress	4 drops
pine	3 drops
cinnamon	3 drops
thyme	2 drops
carrier oil	4 teaspoons (20 ml)

pine	4 drops
juniper berries	4 drops
fennel	4 drops
lime	4 drops
thyme	4 drops
carrier oil	4 teaspoons (20 ml)

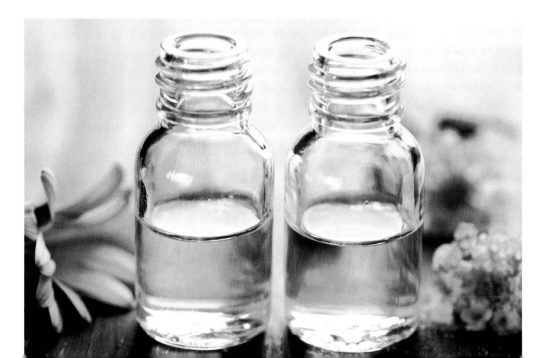

Communication Enhancement

Lack of communication may be the first indication of a troubled relationship. These formulas help encourage the flow of feelings that have been repressed.

Apply the formula to the upper chest, back of the neck, and shoulders.

frankincense	5 drops
benzoin	5 drops
geranium	5 drops
carrier oil	1 tablespoon (15 ml)

frankincense	5 drops
clary sage	5 drops
sandalwood	5 drops
carrier oil	1 tablespoon (15 ml)

spruce	5 drops
pine	5 drops
clary sage	5 drops
carrier oil	1 tablespoon (15 ml)

ylang-ylang	5 drops
pine	5 drops
frankincense	5 drops
carrier oil	1 tablespoon (15 ml)

lemon	5 drops
sandalwood	5 drops
clary sage	5 drops
carrier oil	1 tablespoon (15 ml)

grapefruit	6 drops
spruce	5 drops
patchouli	4 drops
carrier oil	1 tablespoon (15 ml)

Fatigue Relief

Fatigue can result from strenuous physical or mental work, stress, or not getting a restful sleep. Try one of the Sleep Restfully formulas before bedtime. Then, in the morning, apply one of these formulas to energize you.

Massage the blend into the upper chest, back of the neck, shoulders, and down the back.

lime	5 drops		*grapefruit*	6 drops
cumin	5 drops		*palmarosa*	5 drops
clove	5 drops		*thyme*	4 drops
carrier oil	1 tablespoon (15 ml)		*carrier oil*	1 tablespoon (15 ml)

spearmint	6 drops		*bergamot*	5 drops
pine	5 drops		*lemon*	5 drops
ginger	4 drops		*peppermint*	3 drops
carrier oil	1 tablespoon (15 ml)		*carrier oil*	1 tablespoon (15 ml)

rosemary	5 drops		*peppermint*	6 drops
melissa	5 drops		*rosemary*	5 drops
cumin	5 drops		*grapefruit*	4 drops
carrier oil	1 tablespoon (15 ml)		*carrier oil*	1 tablespoon (15 ml)

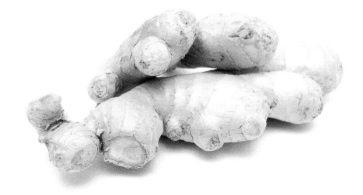

Foot Rejuvenator

To rejuvenate tired and aching feet, try these formulas. Massage the formula from the bottoms of the feet up to the calves.

cajeput	4 drops		lavender	4 drops
lime	4 drops		cajeput	4 drops
rosemary	4 drops		coriander	4 drops
cypress	4 drops		cubeb	4 drops
pine	4 drops		eucalyptus	4 drops
carrier oil	4 teaspoons (20 ml)		carrier oil	4 teaspoons (20 ml)

spearmint	4 drops		grapefruit	4 drops
ginger	4 drops		geranium	4 drops
petitgrain	4 drops		myrtle	3 drops
cypress	3 drops		lime	3 drops
spruce	3 drops		palmarosa	3 drops
eucalyptus	2 drops		thyme	3 drops
carrier oil	4 teaspoons (20 ml)		carrier oil	4 teaspoons (20 ml)

lavender	5 drops		peppermint	5 drops
palmarosa	4 drops		lemon	4 drops
allspice	4 drops		tea tree	4 drops
lemon	4 drops		sage	4 drops
patchouli	3 drops		spruce	3 drops
carrier oil	4 teaspoons (20 ml)		carrier oil	4 teaspoons (20 ml)

Hand Rejuvenator

Massage the formula into both hands, from the fingers to the shoulders.

allspice	5 drops		melissa	5 drops
rosemary	5 drops		cypress	5 drops
peppermint	5 drops		peppermint	5 drops
lavender	5 drops		cinnamon	5 drops
carrier oil	4 teaspoons (20 ml)		carrier oil	4 teaspoons (20 ml)

grapefruit	5 drops		lime	5 drops
lavender	5 drops		thyme	5 drops
spearmint	5 drops		eucalyptus	5 drops
ginger	5 drops		cajeput	5 drops
carrier oil	4 teaspoons (20 ml)		carrier oil	4 teaspoons (20 ml)

lavender	5 drops		geranium	5 drops
spruce	4 drops		grapefruit	4 drops
sweet basil	3 drops		sweet bay	4 drops
lemon	3 drops		black pepper	4 drops
juniper berries	3 drops		guaiacwood	3 drops
allspice	2 drops		carrier oil	4 teaspoons (20 ml)
carrier oil	4 teaspoons (20 ml)			

Mood Elevating

Massage the formula into the upper chest, back of the neck, and shoulders.

palmarosa	4 drops		ylang-ylang	5 drops
ylang-ylang	4 drops		ginger	4 drops
orange	4 drops		patchouli	3 drops
lime	3 drops		bois de rose	3 drops
carrier oil	1 tablespoon (15 ml)		carrier oil	1 tablespoon (15 ml)
rose	5 drops		lemongrass	5 drops
geranium	4 drops		geranium	5 drops
patchouli	4 drops		sweet basil	3 drops
clove	2 drops		lime	2 drops
carrier oil	1 tablespoon (15 ml)		carrier oil	1 tablespoon (15 ml)
melissa	5 drops		frankincense	5 drops
champaca flower	5 drops		ginger	5 drops
lemon	5 drops		grapefruit	5 drops
carrier oil	1 tablespoon (15 ml)		carrier oil	1 tablespoon (15 ml)

ylang-ylang	5 drops		*peppermint*	5 drops
caraway	4 drops		*thyme*	4 drops
sandalwood	4 drops		*grapefruit*	4 drops
cardamom	2 drops		*cypress*	2 drops
carrier oil	1 tablespoon (15 ml)		*carrier oil*	1 tablespoon (15 ml)

Muscle Relaxers

Massage the formula into tight muscles and the surrounding areas.

ginger	10 drops		*geranium*	10 drops
cypress	10 drops		*ginger*	10 drops
black pepper	5 drops		*cypress*	5 drops
juniper berries	5 drops		*juniper berries*	5 drops
sesame	2 tablespoons (30 ml)		*sesame*	2 tablespoons (30 ml)

neroli	9 drops		*ginger*	15 drops
thyme	8 drops		*ylang-ylang*	9 drops
sweet bay	7 drops		*guaiacwood*	6 drops
marjoram	6 drops		*sesame*	2 tablespoons (30 ml)
sesame	2 tablespoons (30 ml)			

For Muscle Soreness

Massage the formula into the specific muscles.

ylang-ylang	5 drops		sweet bay	4 drops
ginger	5 drops		rosemary	4 drops
nutmeg	3 drops		eucalyptus	4 drops
rosemary	2 drops		ylang-ylang	3 drops
carrier oil	1 tablespoon (15 ml)		carrier oil	1 tablespoon (15 ml)

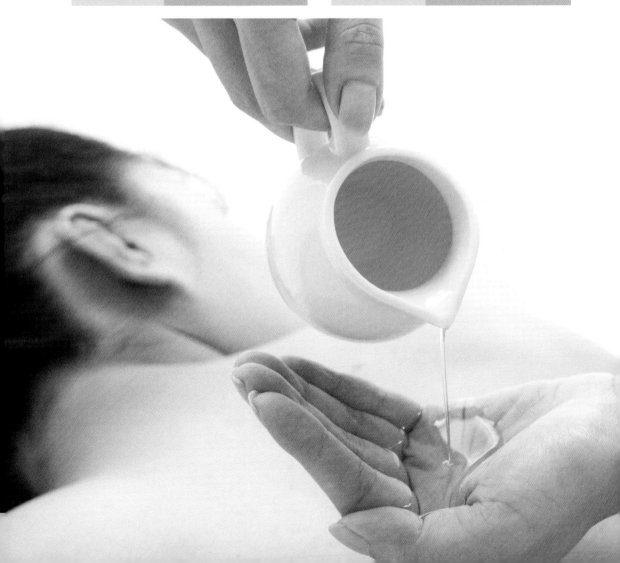

ylang-ylang	4 drops
peppermint	4 drops
thyme	3 drops
ginger	3 drops
lemon	1 drop
carrier oil	1 tablespoon (15 ml)

cinnamon	4 drops
geranium	3 drops
juniper berries	3 drops
lavender	3 drops
peppermint	2 drops
carrier oil	1 tablespoon (15 ml)

allspice	5 drops
cinnamon	4 drops
cajeput	3 drops
chamomile	3 drops
carrier oil	1 tablespoon (15 ml)

grapefruit	5 drops
rose	5 drops
tea tree	3 drops
spearmint	2 drops
carrier oil	1 tablespoon (15 ml)

geranium	5 drops
peppermint	4 drops
marjoram	3 drops
allspice	3 drops
carrier oil	1 tablespoon (15 ml)

spearmint	5 drops
sweet bay	4 drops
benzoin	4 drops
lavender	2 drops
carrier oil	1 tablespoon (15 ml)

Physical Endurance

For centuries, humans have sought ways to increase physical strength and endurance. Whether in hand-to-hand combat or competitive sports, it was advantageous to be as strong as possible.

A simple before-and-after test can be performed by first completing an exercise, such as push-ups, and recording the number accomplished. Then select one of these physical endurance formulas and massage the blend into the specific muscles that were exerted during the exercise. Wait an hour, repeat the exercise, and record the results. After 7 days of daily application, there should be noticeable improvement.

ginger	6 drops		rosemary	5 drops
thyme	5 drops		geranium	5 drops
peppermint	5 drops		grapefruit	5 drops
celery	5 drops		celery	5 drops
grapefruit	5 drops		rose	5 drops
lemon	4 drops		bois de rose	5 drops
grapeseed	2 tablespoons (30 ml)		grapeseed	2 tablespoons (30 ml)

melissa	5 drops		spearmint	6 drops
peppermint	5 drops		cinnamon	5 drops
palmarosa	5 drops		celery	5 drops
allspice	5 drops		bois de rose	5 drops
eucalyptus	4 drops		allspice	5 drops
lime	4 drops		lime	4 drops
ginger	2 drops		borage	1 tablespoon (15 ml)
grapeseed	2 tablespoons (30 ml)		grapeseed	1 tablespoon (15 ml)

ginger	5 drops
myrtle	5 drops
tea tree	5 drops
rose	5 drops
thyme	5 drops
bois de rose	5 drops
grapeseed	2 tablespoons (30 ml)

palmarosa	6 drops
rose	6 drops
eucalyptus	5 drops
cypress	5 drops
spearmint	5 drops
pine	3 drops
grapeseed	2 tablespoons (30 ml)

melissa	5 drops
bois de rose	5 drops
geranium	5 drops
palmarosa	5 drops
spearmint	5 drops
allspice	5 drops
sesame	2 tablespoons (30 ml)

grapefruit	7 drops
cajeput	6 drops
palmarosa	6 drops
rosemary	6 drops
thyme	5 drops
sesame	2 tablespoons (30 ml)

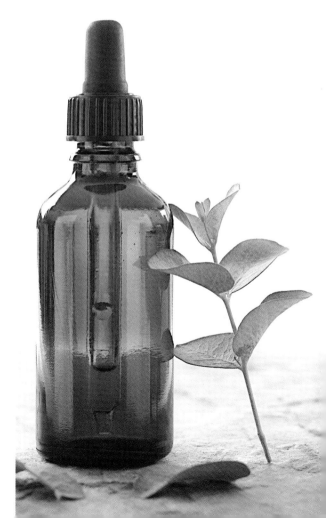

Pre-Event Stress

For those who experience uneasiness or nervous tension before attending an important event or performing, these formulas will help overcome anxiety.

Massage the formula into the back of the neck and shoulders. Use twice—6 hours apart—before the event.

cypress	5 drops
eucalyptus	4 drops
geranium	4 drops
chamomile	3 drops
benzoin	3 drops
lemon	1 drop
carrier oil	4 teaspoons (20 ml)

geranium	5 drops
coriander	3 drops
palmarosa	3 drops
lime	3 drops
neroli	3 drops
lavender	3 drops
carrier oil	4 teaspoons (20 ml)

melissa	5 drops
chamomile	4 drops
fennel	4 drops
cinnamon	3 drops
grapefruit	3 drops
lavender	1 drop
carrier oil	4 teaspoons (20 ml)

allspice	5 drops
basil	3 drops
lime	3 drops
grapefruit	3 drops
cinnamon	3 drops
cubeb	3 drops
carrier oil	4 teaspoons (20 ml)

rose	5 drops
neroli	5 drops
spruce	4 drops
rosemary	3 drops
bois de rose	3 drops
carrier oil	4 teaspoons (20 ml)

sweet bay	5 drops
palmarosa	5 drops
bergamot	4 drops
nutmeg	3 drops
lavender	2 drops
carrier oil	4 teaspoons (20 ml)

bois de rose	5 drops
bergamot	5 drops
neroli	4 drops
mandarin	4 drops
melissa	2 drops
carrier oil	4 teaspoons (20 ml)

geranium	5 drops
melissa	5 drops
petitgrain	5 drops
cypress	5 drops
carrier oil	4 teaspoons (20 ml)

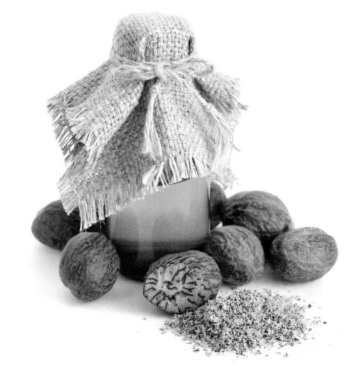

Pre-Game Massage

When you compete in sports, it is important to be at your best. Massaging your muscles before the game will help improve your performance.

sweet bay	5 drops		*bois de rose*	5 drops
allspice	4 drops		*cumin*	5 drops
palmarosa	4 drops		*peppermint*	5 drops
grapefruit	4 drops		*black pepper*	3 drops
eucalyptus	3 drops		*lemon*	2 drops
borage	2 teaspoons (10 ml)		*sesame*	2 teaspoons (10 ml)
flaxseed	2 teaspoons (10 ml)		*grapeseed*	2 teaspoons (10 ml)

grapefruit	5 drops		*allspice*	5 drops
peppermint	5 drops		*eucalyptus*	5 drops
thyme	4 drops		*ginger*	3 drops
nutmeg	3 drops		*black pepper*	3 drops
black pepper	3 drops		*lavender*	2 drops
flaxseed	2 teaspoons (10 ml)		*spearmint*	2 drops
borage	2 teaspoons (10 ml)		*carrier oil*	4 teaspoons (20 ml)

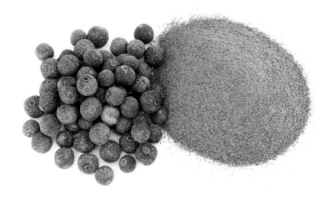

ginger	5 drops	melissa	5 drops
palmarosa	5 drops	lime	5 drops
geranium	4 drops	cypress	4 drops
bois de rose	4 drops	cajeput	4 drops
allspice	2 drops	ginger	2 drops
sesame	4 teaspoons (20 ml)	sesame	4 teaspoons (20 ml)

Premenstrual Syndrome

Before the onset of premenstrual syndrome, massage the blend into the lower back at least once a day.

chamomile	7 drops	rose	10 drops
geranium	7 drops	rosemary	5 drops
lavender	7 drops	grapefruit	5 drops
bois de rose	5 drops	ylang-ylang	5 drops
clary sage	4 drops	cypress	5 drops
borage	1 tablespoon (15 ml)	evening primrose	1 tablespoon (15 ml)
jojoba	1 tablespoon (15 ml)	jojoba	1 tablespoon (15 ml)

ylang-ylang	8 drops	geranium	8 drops
sandalwood	8 drops	bergamot	7 drops
caraway	5 drops	melissa	6 drops
clary sage	5 drops	fennel	4 drops
anise	4 drops	palmarosa	4 drops
sesame	2 tablespoons (30 ml)	flaxseed	2 tablespoons (30 ml)

Premenstrual Syndrome *(continued)*

chamomile	5 drops		caraway	5 drops
allspice	5 drops		sandalwood	5 drops
melissa	5 drops		ylang-ylang	5 drops
bois de rose	5 drops		cumin	5 drops
cypress	5 drops		thyme	5 drops
ginger	5 drops		chamomile	5 drops
sesame	1 tablespoon (15 ml)		evening primrose	1 tablespoon (15 ml)
borage	1 tablespoon (15 ml)		flaxseed	1 tablespoon (15 ml)

rose	10 drops		allspice	7 drops
ylang-ylang	8 drops		neroli	7 drops
bergamot	7 drops		geranium	7 drops
geranium	5 drops		petitgrain	5 drops
sesame	2 tablespoons (30 ml)		benzoin	4 drops
			evening primrose	1 tablespoon (15 ml)
			jojoba	1 tablespoon (15 ml)

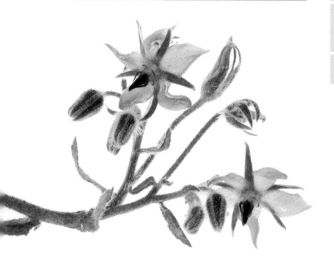

Refreshing

Massage the formula into the back of the neck, the shoulders, and along the back.

spearmint	5 drops		*peppermint*	5 drops
sweet basil	3 drops		*rosemary*	4 drops
lime	3 drops		*clove*	3 drops
rosemary	3 drops		*lime*	3 drops
eucalyptus	3 drops		*lavender*	3 drops
bergamot	3 drops		*sweet basil*	2 drops
carrier oil	4 teaspoons (20 ml)		*carrier oil*	4 teaspoons (20 ml)

pine	5 drops		*grapefruit*	5 drops
geranium	5 drops		*lemon*	5 drops
grapefruit	4 drops		*eucalyptus*	5 drops
peppermint	3 drops		*cajeput*	3 drops
petitgrain	3 drops		*bois de rose*	2 drops
carrier oil	4 teaspoons (20 ml)		*carrier oil*	4 teaspoons (20 ml)

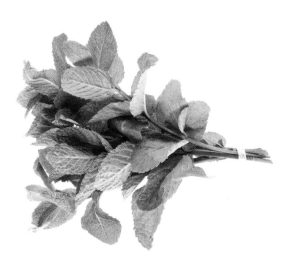

Romance

Make every evening special for you and your partner with your loving touch. For those precious moments, it is important to leave behind the pressures of the world, focus on each other, and enjoy the evening together.

Massage the formula into the back, neck, and shoulders of your partner until the oil is fully absorbed in the skin. This treatment should be mutually reciprocated for best results.

palmarosa	5 drops		*bois de rose*	5 drops
ylang-ylang	5 drops		*cedarwood*	5 drops
patchouli	5 drops		*jasmine*	5 drops
carrier oil	1 tablespoon (15 ml)		*carrier oil*	1 tablespoon (15 ml)

ylang-ylang	4 drops		*rose*	5 drops
clary sage	4 drops		*anise*	4 drops
palmarosa	4 drops		*benzoin*	4 drops
sandalwood	3 drops		*orange*	2 drops
carrier oil	1 tablespoon (15 ml)		*carrier oil*	1 tablespoon (15 ml)

geranium	4 drops		*ylang-ylang*	5 drops
neroli	4 drops		*patchouli*	3 drops
clary sage	3 drops		*clove*	3 drops
palmarosa	3 drops		*orange*	3 drops
anise	1 drop		*clary sage*	1 drop
carrier oil	1 tablespoon (15 ml)		*carrier oil*	1 tablespoon (15 ml)

ylang-ylang	5 drops
mandarin	5 drops
neroli	3 drops
spruce	2 drops
carrier oil	1 tablespoon (15 ml)

sandalwood	5 drops
ylang-ylang	5 drops
black pepper	3 drops
ginger	2 drops
carrier oil	1 tablespoon (15 ml)

Sleep Restfully

Before going to sleep, massage the blend into the upper chest, back of the neck, shoulders, and along the back. Do not drive or do anything that requires full attention after applying these formulas. Good night!

sandalwood	4 drops
marjoram	3 drops
bois de rose	3 drops
chamomile	3 drops
celery	2 drops
carrier oil	1 tablespoon (15 ml)

benzoin	5 drops
sweet basil	3 drops
celery	3 drops
sandalwood	3 drops
lemon	1 drop
carrier oil	1 tablespoon (15 ml)

mandarin	4 drops
lavender	4 drops
neroli	3 drops
lemon	2 drops
dill	2 drops
carrier oil	1 tablespoon (15 ml)

orange	4 drops
anise	3 drops
cedarwood	3 drops
neroli	3 drops
chamomile	2 drops
carrier oil	1 tablespoon (15 ml)

Sleep Restfully *(continued)*

celery	4 drops		petitgrain	5 drops
lavender	4 drops		rose	5 drops
neroli	4 drops		myrtle	3 drops
lemon	3 drops		benzoin	2 drops
carrier oil	1 tablespoon (15 ml)		carrier oil	1 tablespoon (15 ml)

petitgrain	4 drops		vetiver	4 drops
lavender	4 drops		celery	4 drops
lemongrass	4 drops		orange	4 drops
sweet bay	3 drops		sweet basil	3 drops
carrier oil	1 tablespoon (15 ml)		carrier oil	1 tablespoon (15 ml)

spruce	4 drops		dill	4 drops
marjoram	4 drops		celery	4 drops
melissa	4 drops		cedarwood	4 drops
allspice	3 drops		petitgrain	3 drops
carrier oil	1 tablespoon (15 ml)		carrier oil	1 tablespoon (15 ml)

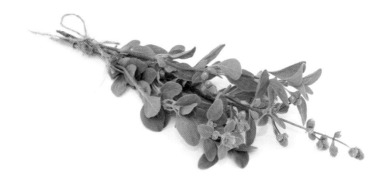

Snoring Remedy

Massage the formula into the upper chest, back of the neck, shoulders, and along the back before going to bed.

bois de rose	4 drops		cajeput	4 drops
geranium	4 drops		myrtle	4 drops
sweet basil	3 drops		marjoram	3 drops
allspice	3 drops		chamomile	3 drops
anise	3 drops		petitgrain	3 drops
lemongrass	3 drops		lavender	3 drops
carrier oil	4 teaspoons (20 ml)		carrier oil	4 teaspoons (20 ml)

cedarwood	4 drops		lavender	5 drops
sweet bay	4 drops		marjoram	4 drops
marjoram	4 drops		myrtle	4 drops
lavender	4 drops		geranium	4 drops
myrtle	4 drops		cajeput	3 drops
carrier oil	4 teaspoons (20 ml)		carrier oil	4 teaspoons (20 ml)

chamomile	4 drops		spruce	5 drops
geranium	4 drops		myrtle	4 drops
cajeput	3 drops		marjoram	3 drops
lavender	3 drops		clary sage	3 drops
grapefruit	3 drops		chamomile	3 drops
cedarwood	3 drops		eucalyptus	2 drops
carrier oil	4 teaspoons (20 ml)		carrier oil	4 teaspoons (20 ml)

For Sprains

Massage the formula into the sprained area. Several applications may be necessary throughout the day, until the painful area feels better.

cypress	5 drops
ylang-ylang	5 drops
lemongrass	5 drops
carrier oil	1 tablespoon (15 ml)

chamomile	5 drops
peppermint	5 drops
cypress	5 drops
carrier oil	1 tablespoon (15 ml)

cajeput	5 drops
lavender	4 drops
celery	4 drops
cypress	2 drops
carrier oil	1 tablespoon (15 ml)

celery	5 drops
lemongrass	5 drops
spearmint	3 drops
eucalyptus	2 drops
carrier oil	1 tablespoon (15 ml)

spearmint	5 drops
marjoram	3 drops
cinnamon	3 drops
lemongrass	3 drops
pine	1 drop
carrier oil	1 tablespoon (15 ml)

lavender	5 drops
peppermint	5 drops
ginger	5 drops
carrier oil	1 tablespoon (15 ml)

Stress Relievers

Massage the formula into the back of the neck, shoulders, along the back, especially the midsection, and any other tense areas.

melissa	5 drops	*bergamot*	5 drops
lavender	5 drops	*mandarin*	4 drops
chamomile	5 drops	*lavender*	4 drops
nutmeg	3 drops	*neroli*	4 drops
benzoin	2 drops	*lemongrass*	3 drops
carrier oil	4 teaspoons (20 ml)	*carrier oil*	4 teaspoons (20 ml)

petitgrain	5 drops	*allspice*	5 drops
chamomile	5 drops	*dill*	4 drops
marjoram	3 drops	*fennel*	3 drops
grapefruit	3 drops	*cinnamon*	3 drops
bois de rose	2 drops	*mandarin*	3 drops
allspice	2 drops	*marjoram*	3 drops
carrier oil	4 teaspoons (20 ml)	*carrier oil*	4 teaspoons (20 ml)

orange	5 drops	*benzoin*	5 drops
bois de rose	5 drops	*petitgrain*	5 drops
petitgrain	5 drops	*eucalyptus*	5 drops
sandalwood	5 drops	*sandalwood*	5 drops
carrier oil	4 teaspoons (20 ml)	*carrier oil*	4 teaspoons (20 ml)

Stress Relievers *(continued)*

allspice	5 drops	cedarwood	4 drops
petitgrain	5 drops	neroli	4 drops
cypress	5 drops	chamomile	4 drops
mandarin	5 drops	melissa	4 drops
carrier oil	4 teaspoons (20 ml)	celery	4 drops
		carrier oil	4 teaspoons (20 ml)

Studying for Exams

To increase alertness and retention of information when you are studying, use one of these formulas.

Before studying, massage the formula into the back of the neck and shoulders. On the day of the exam, apply on a cotton ball the same essential oils used when studying. Place the cotton ball inside a plastic bag and seal tightly. Bring the bag with you and inhale the aromas deeply before and during the exam.

ginger	6 drops	sweet basil	5 drops
grapefruit	5 drops	rosemary	5 drops
juniper berries	4 drops	lemon	5 drops
carrier oil	1 tablespoon (15 ml)	carrier oil	1 tablespoon (15 ml)

bergamot	5 drops	lemon	5 drops
peppermint	5 drops	peppermint	5 drops
cypress	3 drops	sweet basil	3 drops
cinnamon	2 drops	cypress	2 drops
carrier oil	1 tablespoon (15 ml)	carrier oil	1 tablespoon (15 ml)

peppermint	5 drops
clove	5 drops
thyme	5 drops
carrier oil	1 tablespoon (15 ml)

cypress	5 drops
rosemary	5 drops
coriander	5 drops
carrier oil	1 tablespoon (15 ml)

lime	5 drops
rosemary	5 drops
spearmint	5 drops
carrier oil	1 tablespoon (15 ml)

grapefruit	6 drops
petitgrain	5 drops
black pepper	4 drops
carrier oil	1 tablespoon (15 ml)

grapefruit	5 drops
bergamot	5 drops
clove	5 drops
carrier oil	1 tablespoon (15 ml)

lime	5 drops
clove	5 drops
rosemary	3 drops
spearmint	2 drops
carrier oil	1 tablespoon (15 ml)

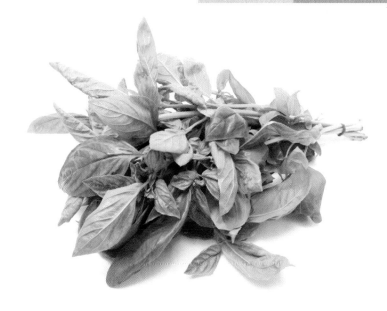

Travel Comfortably

Many people experience discomfort while traveling. These formulas will help you have an enjoyable trip. Massage the formula into the abdomen, chest, back, and shoulders, 1 hour before traveling.

sweet bay	5 drops
peppermint	4 drops
chamomile	4 drops
geranium	4 drops
ginger	3 drops
carrier oil	4 teaspoons (20 ml)

bois de rose	5 drops
ginger	4 drops
dill	4 drops
caraway	4 drops
chamomile	3 drops
carrier oil	4 teaspoons (20 ml)

allspice	5 drops
vetiver	5 drops
lavender	5 drops
caraway	5 drops
carrier oil	4 teaspoons (20 ml)

melissa	5 drops
cypress	5 drops
petitgrain	5 drops
lemongrass	5 drops
carrier oil	4 teaspoons (20 ml)

grapefruit	5 drops
lavender	5 drops
sweet basil	3 drops
thyme	3 drops
clove	3 drops
geranium	1 drop
carrier oil	4 teaspoons (20 ml)

chamomile	5 drops
ginger	4 drops
sandalwood	4 drops
celery	4 drops
neroli	3 drops
carrier oil	4 teaspoons (20 ml)

mandarin	5 drops
lavender	4 drops
juniper berries	4 drops
allspice	4 drops
geranium	3 drops
carrier oil	4 teaspoons (20 ml)

palmarosa	4 drops
neroli	4 drops
allspice	4 drops
cinnamon	4 drops
spearmint	4 drops
carrier oil	4 teaspoons (20 ml)

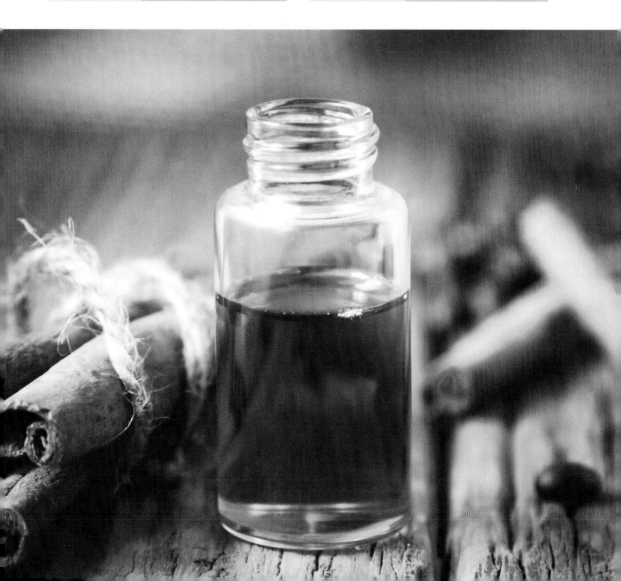

Mist Sprays

Essential oils not only produce a wonderfully scented atmosphere, but they provide a multitude of desirable effects. Refer to Air Fresheners for directions to prepare sprays in this section. For best results, mist over your head about 10 times. With every 2 to 3 sprays, stop and inhale deeply. Be sure to close your eyes to avoid any eye irritation.

Alertness

Many people have difficulty getting going in the morning. To help revitalize the body and feel rejuvenated, use these mists.

peppermint	85 drops		peppermint	60 drops
ginger	40 drops		rosemary	40 drops
grapefruit	35 drops		cypress	40 drops
sweet basil	15 drops		clove	35 drops
pure water	4 fl. oz. (120 ml)		pure water	4 fl. oz. (120 ml)

eucalyptus	30 drops		lime	70 drops
ginger	30 drops		peppermint	45 drops
grapefruit	30 drops		cypress	30 drops
bergamot	30 drops		cinnamon	30 drops
lime	30 drops		pure water	4 fl. oz. (120 ml)
rosemary	25 drops			
pure water	4 fl. oz. (120 ml)			

For Alertness When Driving

There are occasions when a person has to drive while in a fatigued state. Many accidents and injuries are caused by drivers who fall asleep at the wheel. If you are very tired, do not drive, but if you must drive, spray one of these mists in your car to help you stay awake. Be especially careful not to spray any mist near your eyes.

peppermint	110 drops		peppermint	80 drops
cinnamon	35 drops		thyme	40 drops
lime	35 drops		rosemary	40 drops
patchouli	20 drops		grapefruit	40 drops
pure water	4 fl. oz. (120 ml)		pure water	4 fl. oz. (120 ml)

lime	75 drops		pine	60 drops
rosemary	50 drops		lemon	60 drops
clove	45 drops		rosemary	60 drops
peppermint	30 drops		sage	20 drops
pure water	4 fl. oz. (120 ml)		pure water	4 fl. oz. (120 ml)

rosemary	50 drops		pine	50 drops
lemon	50 drops		thyme	40 drops
cinnamon	50 drops		spearmint	40 drops
geranium	25 drops		cumin	25 drops
cypress	25 drops		juniper berries	25 drops
pure water	4 fl. oz. (120 ml)		clove	20 drops
			pure water	4 fl. oz. (120 ml)

For Alertness When Driving (continued)

peppermint	80 drops		spearmint	120 drops
lime	75 drops		cypress	40 drops
rosemary	45 drops		lemon	40 drops
pure water	4 fl. oz. (120 ml)		pure water	4 fl. oz. (120 ml)

Alertness When Studying

To increase alertness and retention of information, mist numerous times while studying and inhale deeply. On the day of the exam, apply a few drops of each essential oil to a cotton ball from the mist formula used when studying. Place the cotton ball inside a plastic bag and seal tightly. Bring the bag with you, and inhale the aromas deeply before and during the exam.

lime	80 drops		clove	50 drops
rosemary	60 drops		pine	50 drops
ginger	20 drops		spearmint	50 drops
sweet basil	15 drops		lemon	25 drops
pure water	4 fl. oz. (120 ml)		pure water	4 fl. oz. (120 ml)

lemon	70 drops		grapefruit	50 drops
peppermint	45 drops		clove	40 drops
petitgrain	20 drops		sweet basil	30 drops
clove	20 drops		bergamot	30 drops
thyme	20 drops		ginger	25 drops
pure water	4 fl. oz. (120 ml)		pure water	4 fl. oz. (120 ml)

bergamot	40 drops		spearmint	40 drops
grapefruit	40 drops		lemon	40 drops
peppermint	40 drops		lavender	30 drops
juniper berries	30 drops		eucalyptus	25 drops
lavender	25 drops		rosemary	25 drops
pure water	4 fl. oz. (120 ml)		sweet basil	15 drops
			pure water	4 fl. oz. (120 ml)

Breathe More Easily During Aerobics, Sports, and Other Exercise

Vigorous exercise strains the respiratory system. Before exercising, spray these mists into the air and breathe deeply to help soothe breathing passages.

peppermint	40 drops		lime	50 drops
eucalyptus	40 drops		pine	40 drops
cajeput	40 drops		tea tree	30 drops
lemon	30 drops		cubeb	30 drops
pure water	4 fl. oz. (120 ml)		pure water	4 fl. oz. (120 ml)

spruce	40 drops		cedarwood	40 drops
lavender	40 drops		cajeput	40 drops
spearmint	35 drops		lavender	40 drops
eucalyptus	35 drops		myrtle	30 drops
pure water	4 fl. oz. (120 ml)		pure water	4 fl. oz. (120 ml)

Breathe More Easily During Aerobics, Sports, and Other Exercise *(continued)*

lime	50 drops
lavender	50 drops
eucalyptus	30 drops
clove	20 drops
pure water	4 fl. oz. (120 ml)

myrtle	40 drops
lemon	40 drops
pine	40 drops
lemongrass	30 drops
pure water	4 fl. oz. (120 ml)

myrtle	30 drops
cajeput	30 drops
eucalyptus	30 drops
clove	30 drops
lime	30 drops
pure water	4 fl. oz. (120 ml)

peppermint	40 drops
rosemary	30 drops
lime	30 drops
lavender	30 drops
marjoram	20 drops
pure water	4 fl. oz. (120 ml)

lavender	50 drops
cajeput	30 drops
grapefruit	20 drops
clove	20 drops
spruce	20 drops
thyme	10 drops
pure water	4 fl. oz. (120 ml)

pine	40 drops
spruce	40 drops
grapefruit	40 drops
lavender	30 drops
pure water	4 fl. oz. (120 ml)

Breathe More Easily in Stuffy Rooms

rosemary	30 drops		lemongrass	30 drops
geranium	30 drops		spruce	30 drops
spruce	25 drops		myrtle	30 drops
thyme	25 drops		lime	30 drops
lime	25 drops		allspice	15 drops
cedarwood	15 drops		lavender	15 drops
pure water	4 fl. oz. (120 ml)		pure water	4 fl. oz. (120 ml)

spearmint	30 drops		eucalyptus	40 drops
pine	25 drops		lemon	40 drops
juniper berries	20 drops		cypress	25 drops
lemon	20 drops		lavender	25 drops
cajeput	20 drops		grapefruit	20 drops
lavender	20 drops		pure water	4 fl. oz. (120 ml)
myrtle	15 drops			
pure water	4 fl. oz. (120 ml)			

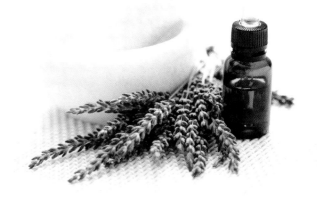

Calming

allspice	45 drops		spruce	40 drops
dill	25 drops		lavender	40 drops
orange	25 drops		geranium	20 drops
Peru balsam	25 drops		petitgrain	20 drops
fennel	15 drops		cedarwood	20 drops
cinnamon	15 drops		lemon	10 drops
pure water	4 fl. oz. (120 ml)		pure water	4 fl. oz. (120 ml)

lemongrass	35 drops		ylang-ylang	40 drops
anise	25 drops		orange	30 drops
allspice	25 drops		chamomile	25 drops
mandarin	25 drops		benzoin	25 drops
vetiver	20 drops		bois de rose	15 drops
bergamot	20 drops		melissa	15 drops
pure water	4 fl. oz. (120 ml)		pure water	4 fl. oz. (120 ml)

marjoram	30 drops		mandarin	60 drops
cajeput	30 drops		lavender	50 drops
lavender	30 drops		bois de rose	20 drops
petitgrain	30 drops		petitgrain	20 drops
vetiver	30 drops		pure water	4 fl. oz. (120 ml)
pure water	4 fl. oz. (120 ml)			

Calming for Overactive Children

Mist the spray into the air several times.

mandarin	40 drops	allspice	30 drops
marjoram	30 drops	chamomile	30 drops
lavender	30 drops	mandarin	30 drops
cedarwood	20 drops	vetiver	30 drops
pure water	4 fl. oz. (120 ml)	pure water	4 fl. oz. (120 ml)

Calming for Dogs

Mist the spray into the air several times.

marjoram	60 drops	lavender	50 drops
lavender	40 drops	chamomile	50 drops
orange	20 drops	mandarin	20 drops
pure water	4 fl. oz. (120 ml)	pure water	4 fl. oz. (120 ml)

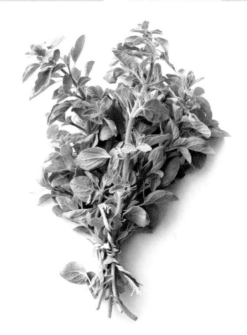

Colds & Flu

Use the mist spray numerous times during the day as needed.

Please note: Colloidal silver is optional to add to these formulas. If it is included in the mist, please only use distilled water. If the colloidal silver is not being used, pure filtered water such as that produced by reverse osmosis is fine.

distilled water	2 fl. oz. (60 ml)
lemon	25 drops
clove	25 drops
sage	25 drops
colloidal silver	10 drops (optional)

distilled water	2 fl. oz. (60 ml)
spruce	30 drops
spearmint	30 drops
vetiver	15 drops
colloidal silver	10 drops (optional)

distilled water	2 fl. oz. (60 ml)
peppermint	25 drops
clove	25 drops
lemon	13 drops
ginger	12 drops
colloidal silver	10 drops (optional)

distilled water	2 fl. oz. (60 ml)
marjoram	25 drops
guaiacwood	25 drops
cinnamon	13 drops
grapefruit	12 drops
colloidal silver	10 drops (optional)

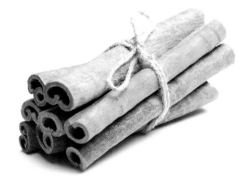

distilled water	2 fl. oz. (60 ml)		distilled water	2 fl. oz. (60 ml)
peppermint	30 drops		spearmint	25 drops
sage	15 drops		sage	25 drops
cinnamon	15 drops		marjoram	25 drops
clove	15 drops		colloidal silver	10 drops (optional)
colloidal silver	10 drops (optional)			

Holiday Atmosphere

allspice	30 drops		clove	40 drops
dill	30 drops		cinnamon	30 drops
caraway	30 drops		ginger	30 drops
clove	30 drops		orange	20 drops
pure water	4 fl. oz. (120 ml)		pure water	4 fl. oz. (120 ml)

spruce	75 drops		cypress	40 drops
cedarwood	25 drops		pine	30 drops
juniper berries	25 drops		eucalyptus	30 drops
pure water	4 fl. oz. (120 ml)		sandalwood	20 drops
			pure water	4 fl. oz. (120 ml)

Mood Elevating

bergamot	60 drops	*spearmint*	60 drops
lime	50 drops	*clove*	40 drops
geranium	20 drops	*grapefruit*	30 drops
ylang-ylang	20 drops	*tolu balsam*	20 drops
pure water	4 fl. oz. (120 ml)	*pure water*	4 fl. oz. (120 ml)

bois de rose	50 drops	*melissa*	30 drops
lemon	35 drops	*lemongrass*	30 drops
melissa	35 drops	*ylang-ylang*	30 drops
geranium	30 drops	*benzoin*	20 drops
pure water	4 fl. oz. (120 ml)	*clove*	20 drops
		cumin	20 drops
		pure water	4 fl. oz. (120 ml)

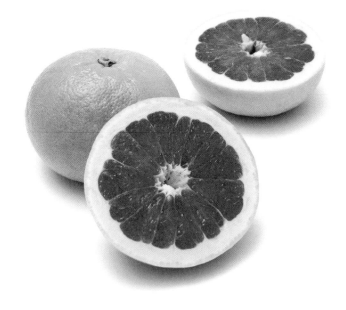

Premenstrual Syndrome

It has been estimated that nearly 90 percent of women suffer from premenstrual syndrome (PMS) sometime in their lives. The syndrome's effects range from outright violence to mild depression to crying spells. These mists can help elevate the mood and make PMS bearable. Spray many times during the day, and inhale the mist deeply.

bergamot	60 drops
geranium	60 drops
allspice	40 drops
anise	30 drops
patchouli	10 drops
pure water	4 fl. oz. (120 ml)

cypress	50 drops
neroli	50 drops
bergamot	40 drops
orange	30 drops
allspice	30 drops
pure water	4 fl. oz. (120 ml)

ylang-ylang	35 drops
bergamot	35 drops
sandalwood	35 drops
lime	35 drops
palmarosa	30 drops
caraway	30 drops
pure water	4 fl. oz. (120 ml)

lemongrass	50 drops
cypress	40 drops
fennel	30 drops
lavender	30 drops
geranium	30 drops
caraway	20 drops
pure water	4 fl. oz. (120 ml)

Premenstrual Syndrome *(continued)*

chamomile	40 drops		petitgrain	60 drops
lavender	40 drops		ylang-ylang	50 drops
lemon	40 drops		grapefruit	40 drops
geranium	40 drops		bergamot	30 drops
caraway	40 drops		fennel	20 drops
pure water	4 fl. oz. (120 ml)		pure water	4 fl. oz. (120 ml)

neroli	40 drops		geranium	60 drops
jasmine	30 drops		melissa	60 drops
geranium	30 drops		grapefruit	40 drops
palmarosa	30 drops		allspice	40 drops
lime	30 drops		pure water	4 fl. oz. (120 ml)
allspice	30 drops			
pure water	4 fl. oz. (120 ml)			

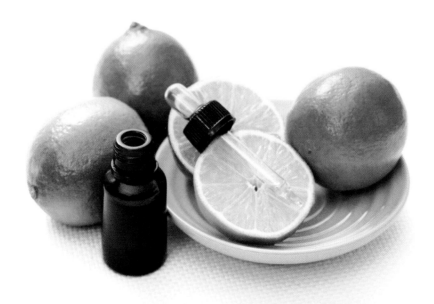

Refreshing

lime	90 drops		lemon	50 drops
peppermint	50 drops		cypress	50 drops
eucalyptus	10 drops		clove	50 drops
pure water	4 fl. oz. (120 ml)		pure water	4 fl. oz. (120 ml)

grapefruit	40 drops		grapefruit	50 drops
petitgrain	40 drops		lemon	50 drops
peppermint	40 drops		spearmint	50 drops
lime	30 drops		pure water	4 fl. oz. (120 ml)
pure water	4 fl. oz. (120 ml)			

Room Disinfectant

tea tree	65 drops		lavender	70 drops
thyme	50 drops		allspice	40 drops
eucalyptus	35 drops		cinnamon	40 drops
pure water	4 fl. oz. (120 ml)		pure water	4 fl. oz. (120 ml)

clove	75 drops		cinnamon	65 drops
lavender	45 drops		patchouli	45 drops
bergamot	30 drops		lemongrass	40 drops
pure water	4 fl. oz. (120 ml)		pure water	4 fl. oz. (120 ml)

Sauna/Steam Room

Spray the mist away from your body so that when you perspire the spray does not come in contact with your eyes.

eucalyptus	30 drops
tea tree	30 drops
pine	30 drops
lavender	30 drops
pure water	4 fl. oz. (120 ml)

lavender	50 drops
cajeput	25 drops
spruce	25 drops
eucalyptus	20 drops
pure water	4 fl. oz. (120 ml)

peppermint	30 drops
lavender	30 drops
cedarwood	30 drops
spruce	15 drops
eucalyptus	15 drops
pure water	4 fl. oz. (120 ml)

sandalwood	60 drops
spearmint	60 drops
pure water	4 fl. oz. (120 ml)

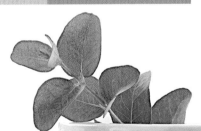

Snoring Remedy

Mist numerous times before going to sleep and have the snorer inhale deeply. If necessary, mist again during the night to quiet the snorer.

geranium	50 drops
lavender	50 drops
marjoram	50 drops
cedarwood	20 drops
eucalyptus	15 drops
sweet basil	15 drops
pure water	4 fl. oz. (120 ml)

spruce	55 drops
myrtle	45 drops
eucalyptus	30 drops
sweet bay	30 drops
grapefruit	20 drops
marjoram	20 drops
pure water	4 fl. oz. (120 ml)

spruce	35 drops
lavender	35 drops
anise	35 drops
sandalwood	35 drops
cubeb	30 drops
lemongrass	30 drops
pure water	4 fl. oz. (120 ml)

dill	40 drops
tea tree	40 drops
orange	30 drops
lemongrass	30 drops
allspice	30 drops
marjoram	30 drops
pure water	4 fl. oz. (120 ml)

Snoring Remedy *(continued)*

marjoram	60 drops		cajeput	55 drops
lemongrass	40 drops		allspice	55 drops
sandalwood	40 drops		lavender	50 drops
myrtle	30 drops		grapefruit	20 drops
lavender	30 drops		celery	20 drops
pure water	4 fl. oz. (120 ml)		pure water	4 fl. oz. (120 ml)

Stress Relievers

cypress	50 drops		melissa	70 drops
lemongrass	40 drops		fennel	20 drops
lavender	20 drops		cinnamon	20 drops
clove	20 drops		chamomile	20 drops
patchouli	20 drops		lavender	20 drops
pure water	4 fl. oz. (120 ml)		pure water	4 fl. oz. (120 ml)

lemon	40 drops		petitgrain	40 drops
sandalwood	40 drops		mandarin	40 drops
allspice	40 drops		lemongrass	40 drops
bois de rose	30 drops		palmarosa	30 drops
pure water	4 fl. oz. (120 ml)		pure water	4 fl. oz. (120 ml)

chamomile	60 drops
geranium	30 drops
coriander	30 drops
lavender	30 drops
pure water	4 fl. oz. (120 ml)

allspice	50 drops
mandarin	50 drops
patchouli	20 drops
melissa	20 drops
pure water	4 fl. oz. (120 ml)

grapefruit	50 drops
mandarin	35 drops
allspice	35 drops
benzoin	30 drops
pure water	4 fl. oz. (120 ml)

lemon	45 drops
dill	40 drops
palmarosa	35 drops
ylang-ylang	30 drops
pure water	4 fl. oz. (120 ml)

Travel Comfortably

Many people experience discomfort when traveling. These mists will soothe the stomach and help make traveling more enjoyable. Use before and during the trip, as necessary. Inhale deeply.

caraway	35 drops
melissa	35 drops
lemongrass	30 drops
geranium	25 drops
lavender	25 drops
cinnamon	25 drops
pure water	4 fl. oz. (120 ml)

chamomile	35 drops
lemon	35 drops
sweet bay	30 drops
lavender	25 drops
ginger	25 drops
cinnamon	25 drops
pure water	4 fl. oz. (120 ml)

Travel Comfortably *(continued)*

cypress	45 drops		ginger	30 drops
melissa	45 drops		allspice	30 drops
chamomile	40 drops		cinnamon	30 drops
fennel	25 drops		geranium	30 drops
ginger	20 drops		cardamom	30 drops
pure water	4 fl. oz. (120 ml)		pure water	4 fl. oz. (120 ml)

spearmint	50 drops		caraway	45 drops
melissa	45 drops		peppermint	30 drops
cinnamon	30 drops		thyme	30 drops
lemongrass	20 drops		nutmeg	20 drops
cypress	20 drops		fennel	20 drops
allspice	10 drops		marjoram	15 drops
pure water	4 fl. oz. (120 ml)		allspice	15 drops
			pure water	4 fl. oz. (120 ml)

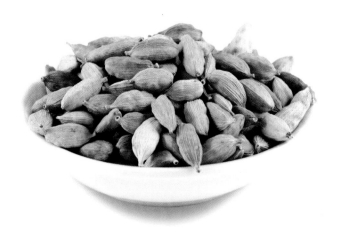

Mouthwash

For fresh breath, use one of these mouthwashes.

Measure and then pour purified water in a glass bottle. Add the essential oils, honey, and two pinches of unrefined sea salt (optional), warm the water to melt the honey, stir well, and rinse your mouth and throat. Cap the bottle, label it, and store for a later use.

pure water	8 fl. oz. (120 ml)		pure water	8 fl. oz. (120 ml)
honey	2 teaspoons (10 ml)		honey	2 teaspoons (10 ml)
clove	6 drops		anise	6 drops
orange	6 drops		lemon	6 drops
sea salt	2 pinches (optional)		sea salt	2 pinches (optional)

pure water	8 fl. oz. (120 ml)		pure water	8 fl. oz. (120 ml)
honey	2 teaspoons (10 ml)		honey	2 teaspoons (10 ml)
spearmint	8 drops		spearmint	6 drops
sandalwood	4 drops		orange	6 drops
sea salt	2 pinches (optional)		sea salt	2 pinches (optional)

pure water	8 fl. oz. (120 ml)		pure water	8 fl. oz. (120 ml)
honey	2 teaspoons (10 ml)		honey	2 teaspoons (10 ml)
cinnamon	6 drops		lemon	6 drops
orange	6 drops		tangerine	6 drops
sea salt	2 pinches (optional)		sea salt	2 pinches (optional)

Potpourri

Making your own potpourri is a wonderful way to add a scent your home. Gather dried leaves, flowers, and small wood shavings. Crush these plant materials to the desired size. Place ½ cup (120 ml) of plant material in a wide-mouthed glass jar, and add the essential oil formula. Stir the contents well and tighten the lid on the jar. Let the potpourri sit for several days to allow the aroma molecules to be absorbed by the plant material.

Citrus Scent

grapefruit	80 drops	lime	100 drops
lemon	50 drops	orange	40 drops
clove	50 drops	cinnamon	30 drops
benzoin	20 drops	patchouli	30 drops

Floral Scent

ylang-ylang	70 drops	bois de rose	50 drops
geranium	50 drops	ylang-ylang	50 drops
orange	50 drops	lemon	30 drops
clove	20 drops	clove	30 drops
benzoin	10 drops	cedarwood	20 drops

Forest Scent

spruce	100 drops	eucalyptus	50 drops
lavender	30 drops	myrtle	50 drops
clove	30 drops	cajeput	50 drops
rosemary	30 drops	juniper berries	30 drops
patchouli	10 drops	Peru balsam	20 drops

Minty Scent

spearmint	100 drops	peppermint	110 drops
lemon	50 drops	rosemary	30 drops
petitgrain	20 drops	grapefruit	30 drops
peppermint	20 drops	benzoin	30 drops
benzoin	10 drops		

Spicy Scent

caraway	75 drops	cinnamon	75 drops
clove	75 drops	allspice	75 drops
cumin	30 drops	anise	40 drops
patchouli	20 drops	benzoin	10 drops

Pre-Shave

Mix the oils together well, and apply them to the area before shaving.

flaxseed	20 drops	flaxseed	20 drops
lavender	3 drops	bois de rose	2 drops
allspice	1 drop	allspice	1 drop

flaxseed	20 drops	flaxseed	20 drops
geranium	2 drops	lavender	2 drops
sweet bay	1 drop	chamomile	1 drop

Skin Care

The skin is a very resilient organ of the body. After being scraped, cut, burned, or scratched, it can miraculously heal itself fairly quickly. If treated properly, the skin will show little sign of wear and tear over the years.

Combine all ingredients from the formula to help rejuvenate your skin. Before using, wash your skin thoroughly, then massage in a portion of the formula. Apply daily.

Normal Skin

chamomile	10 drops		lavender	10 drops
bois de rose	10 drops		palmarosa	10 drops
benzoin	10 drops		geranium	10 drops
hazelnut	2 tablespoons (30 ml)		hazelnut	2 tablespoons (30 ml)

lavender	10 drops		rose	10 drops
chamomile	5 drops		frankincense	10 drops
fennel	5 drops		jasmine	10 drops
benzoin	5 drops		hazelnut	2 tablespoons (30 ml)
geranium	5 drops			
hazelnut	2 tablespoons (30 ml)			

Dry Skin

benzoin	10 drops		sandalwood	10 drops
rosemary	8 drops		bois de rose	10 drops
geranium	8 drops		lavender	10 drops
lavender	4 drops		avocado	2 tablespoons (30 ml)
flaxseed	2 tablespoons (30 ml)			

patchouli	10 drops		*chamomile*	10 drops
palmarosa	10 drops		*lavender*	10 drops
geranium	10 drops		*palmarosa*	10 drops
jojoba	2 tablespoons (30 ml)		*sesame*	2 tablespoons (30 ml)

Oily Skin

ylang-ylang	10 drops		*lime*	15 drops
lemon	10 drops		*cypress*	5 drops
cypress	5 drops		*ylang-ylang*	5 drops
petitgrain	5 drops		*juniper berries*	5 drops
grapeseed	2 tablespoons (30 ml)		*grapeseed*	2 tablespoons (30 ml)

ylang-ylang	8 drops		*orange*	10 drops
juniper berries	8 drops		*lemon*	10 drops
orange	8 drops		*petitgrain*	10 drops
lavender	6 drops		*grapeseed*	2 tablespoons (30 ml)
grapeseed	2 tablespoons (30 ml)			

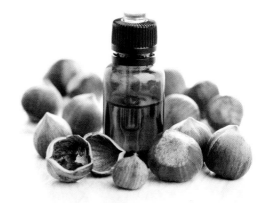

Problem Skin

myrrh	10 drops		myrrh	10 drops
chamomile	10 drops		palmarosa	10 drops
bois de rose	5 drops		frankincense	10 drops
lavender	5 drops		borage	1 tablespoon (15 ml)
kukui nut	2 tablespoons (30 ml)		flaxseed	1 tablespoon (15 ml)

myrrh	15 drops		sandalwood	10 drops
patchouli	10 drops		lavender	10 drops
geranium	5 drops		bois de rose	10 drops
borage	1 tablespoon (15 ml)		sesame	1 tablespoon (15 ml)
kukui nut	1 tablespoon (15 ml)		flaxseed	1 tablespoon (15 ml)

lavender	20 drops		chamomile	15 drops
palmarosa	10 drops		bois de rose	15 drops
evening primrose	1 tablespoon (15 ml)		sesame	1 tablespoon (15 ml)
flaxseed	1 tablespoon (15 ml)		kukui nut	1 tablespoon (15 ml)

petitigrain	10 drops		myrrh	10 drops
benzoin	10 drops		lavender	10 drops
tea tree	10 drops		benzoin	10 drops
evening primrose	1 tablespoon (15 ml)		borage	1 tablespoon (15 ml)
kukui nut	1 tablespoon (15 ml)		walnut	1 tablespoon (15 ml)

Steam Inhalation

Add 5 to 10 drops of essential oil to a bowl of hot water. Drape a towel over the head, close your eyes, and inhale the vapors. Select from the following oils.

cajeput	lemongrass	peppermint	spearmint
eucalyptus	marjoram	pine	spruce
lavender	myrtle	rosemary	tea tree

Sunburn Relief

Gently apply the formula on the sunburned area, several times a day.

lavender	3 drops		chamomile	3 drops
chamomile	2 drops		geranium	2 drops
aloe vera gel	1 teaspoon (5 ml)		sweet almond	1 teaspoon (5 ml)

lavender	5 drops		lavender	5 drops
aloe vera gel	1 teaspoon (5 ml)		avocado	1 teaspoon (5 ml)

Suntan Oil

Many people avoid being outdoors because of the discomfort of getting sunburned. With this jojoba and sesame suntan oil, you will get a wonderful tan. First apply jojoba oil on the entire skin area that will be exposed to the sun. Then rub sesame oil over the same area.

jojoba	(to cover area)
sesame	(to cover area)

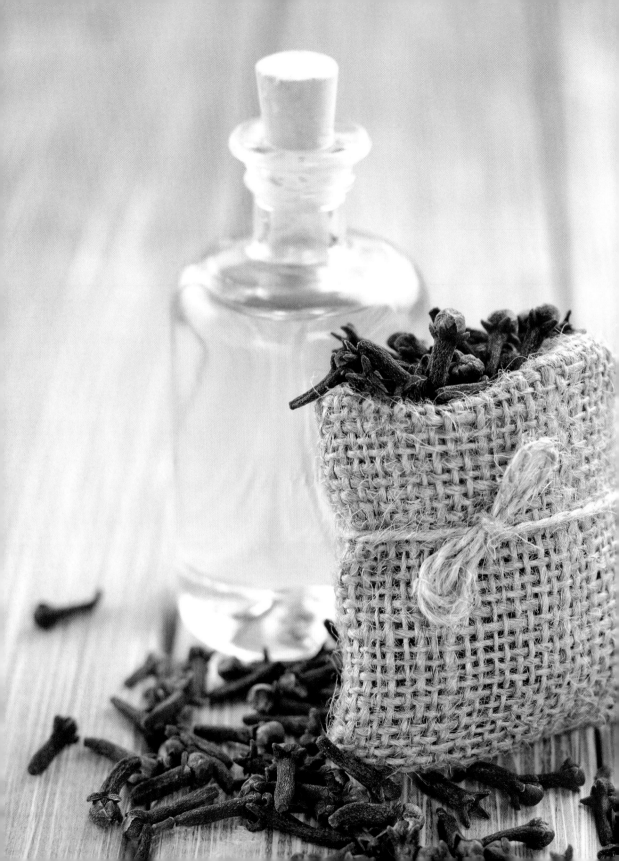

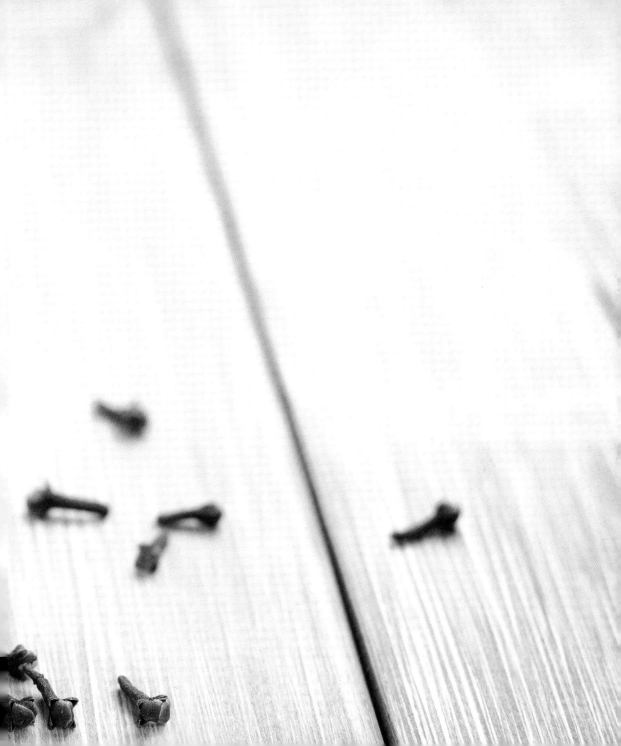

CARRIER OILS

Carrier oils play a key role by diluting essential oils for use in massage, skin, and hair care blends. These oils are beneficial in protecting the skin by moisturizing, soothing, softening, and nourishing the skin cells as the oils are absorbed deep into the skin layers. Whenever essential oils are applied topically, carrier oils must be combined with them to form a blend.

Almond (Sweet)

Prunus amygdalus, Prunus dulcis

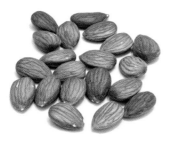

Uses

Massage oil; skin and hair care; moisturizing to the skin; suntanning oil

Avocado

Persea americana, Persea gratissima

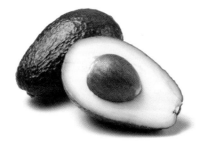

Uses

Massage oil; skin and hair care; moisturizing; removes impurities from the skin

Borage

Borago officianalis

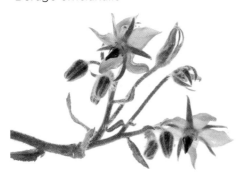

Uses

Calming; helps premenstrual stress; relieves menstrual pain; reduces inflammation; massage oil; skin care; inflamed skin

Flaxseed

Linum usitatissimum

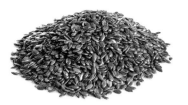

Uses

Massage oil; skin care

Grapeseed

Vitis vinifera

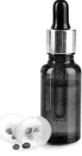

Uses

Massage oil; general skin care

Hazelnut

Corylus avellana

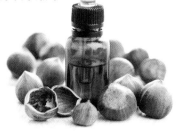

Uses

Massage oil; skin care; moisturizes, softens, and repairs dry and damaged skin

Jojoba

Simmondsia chinensis

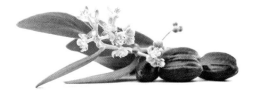

Uses

Massage oil; skin, hair, and scalp care; moisturizes and softens dry skin; helps with stretch marks; suntanning oil for those who burn easily in the sun

Kukui Nut

Aleurites moluccana

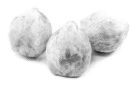

Uses

Massage oil; skin care; balances, rejuvenates, and softens the skin

Macadamia Nut

Macadamia integrifolia, Macadamia ternifolia, Macadamia tetraphylla

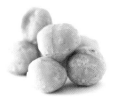

Uses

Massage oil; skin care; softens and restores the skin

Olive

Olea europaea

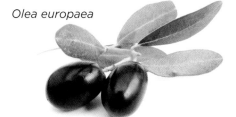

Uses

Massage oil; skin care

Sesame

Sesamum indicum, Sesamum orientale

Uses

Massage oil; skin, hair, and scalp care; moisturizing and soothing to the skin

Shea Butter

Butyrospermum parkii

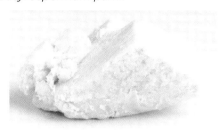

Uses

Skin and hair moisturizer; suntan cream

Walnut

Juglans regia

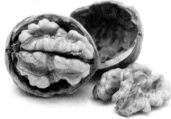

Uses

Massage oil; skin care

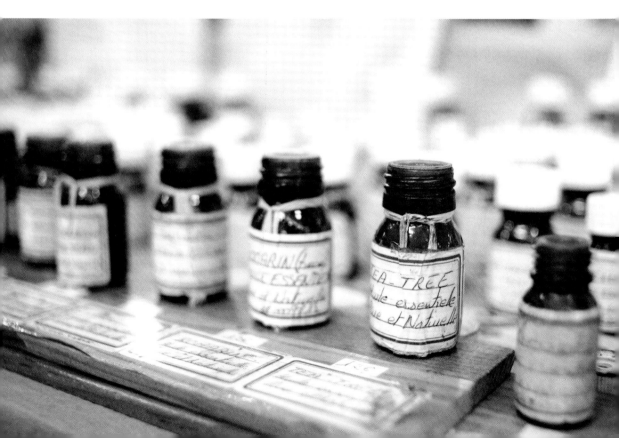

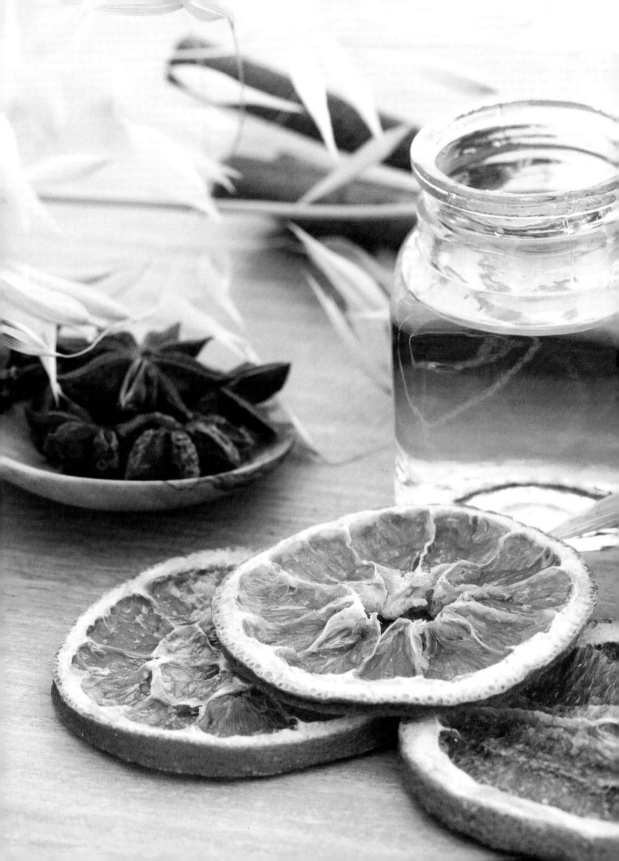

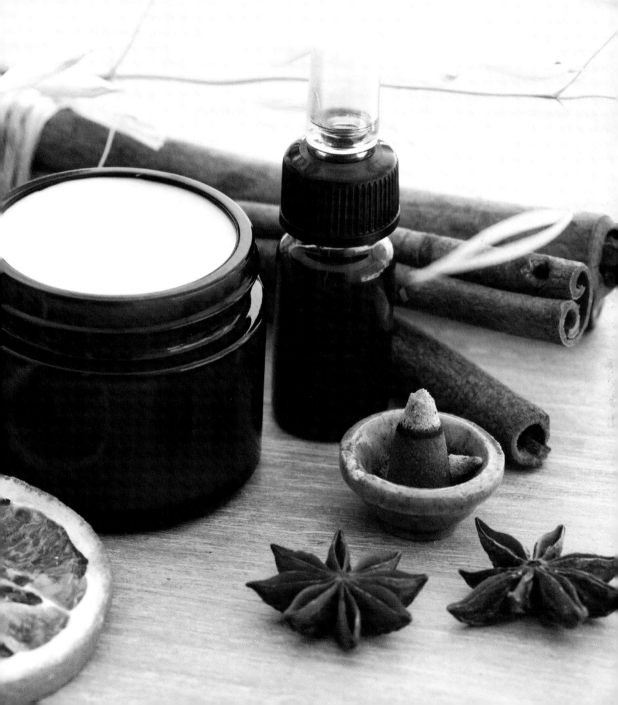

ESSENTIAL OILS
A TO Z

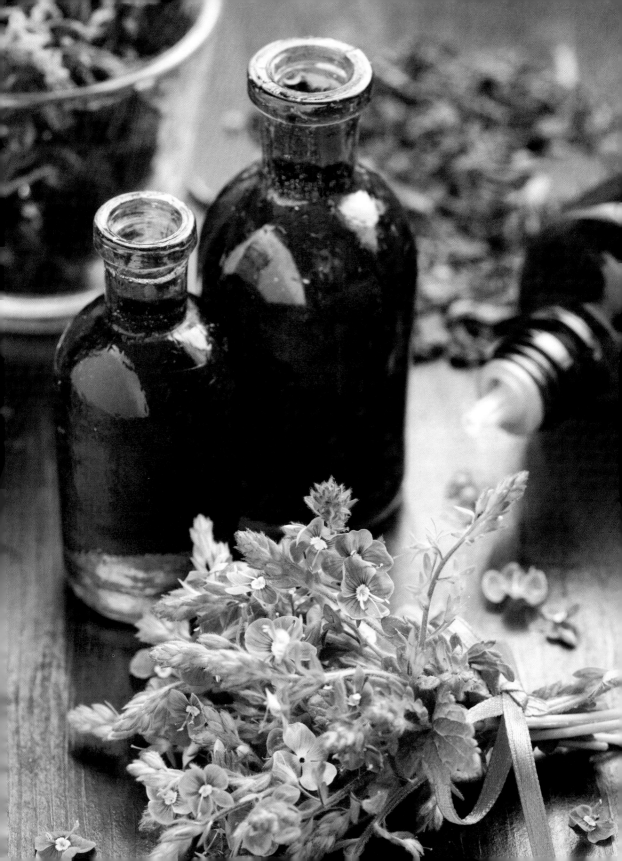

Allspice (Pimento)

Pimenta officianalis

Scent: clove

Uses

Warming to the body; reduces stress; calming; relaxes tight muscles; lessens pain; promotes restful sleep; mood uplifting; vapors help breathing; improves digestion; disinfectant

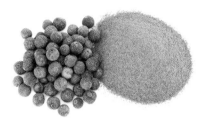

Aloe

Aloe vera or *Aloe barbadensis*

Uses

Lessens pain; healing, moisturizing, rejuvenating for skin; hydrates dry hair

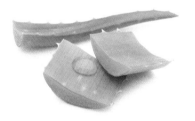

Anise

Pimpinella anisum

Scent: licorice

Uses

Calming; lessens pain; aphrodisiac; promotes restful sleep; vapors help breathing; improves digestion; increases appetite; stimulates lactation in nursing mothers

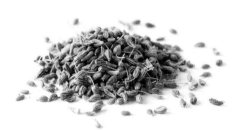

(Sweet) Basil

Ocimum basilicum

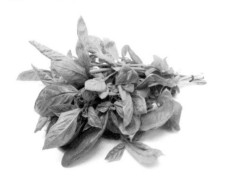

Scent: Slightly licorice

Uses

Calming; lessens pain; promotes restful sleep; mood uplifting; helps relieve fatigue; improves digestion; stimulates lactation in nursing mothers; improves mental clarity and memory; helps reduce cellulite deposits; soothes insect bites

---

(Sweet) Bay

Laurus nobilis

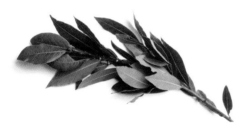

Scent: Spicy

Uses

Relaxes tight muscles; soothes sprains lessens pain; calming; promotes restful sleep; vapors help breathing; improves digestion; improves mental clarity and memory; promotes perspiration; disinfectant; repels insects

---

Benzoin

Styrax benzoin

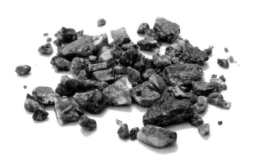

Scent: Cinnamon-vanilla

Uses

Warming to the body; reduces stress; calming; helpful for meditation; relaxes tight muscles; breaks up congestion; reduces inflammation; promotes restful sleep; mood uplifting; helps reduce cellulite deposits; healing to the skin; preservative in cosmetics; fixative for perfumes and fragrances

Bergamot

Citrus bergamia

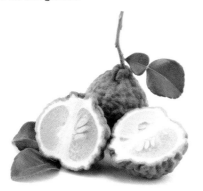

Scent: Citrus

Uses

Reduces anxiety, nervous tension, and stress; balances nervous system; mood uplifting; helps relieve fatigue; disinfectant

Bois de Rose (Rosewood)

Aniba rosaeodora

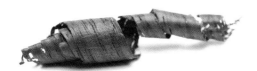

Scent: Slightly rosy

Uses

Relieves nervousness and stress; calming; lessens pain; promotes restful sleep; mood uplifting; skin tissue regenerator and moisturizer

Cajeput

Melaleuca leucadendron

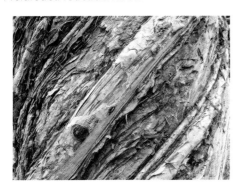

Scent: Camphor

Uses

Slightly warming to the body; calming; relaxes tight muscles; relieves muscle aches and pains; promotes restful sleep; breaks up congestion; vapors help breathing; disinfectant; repels insects

Caraway

Carum carvi

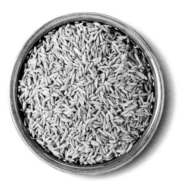

Scent: Spicy

Uses

Relieves pain; vapors help breathing; improves digestion; increases appetite; stimulates lactation in nursing mothers

Cardamom

Elettaria cardamomum

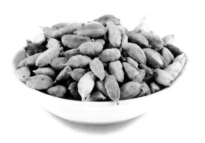

Scent: Spicy

Uses

Warming to the body; relieves pain; mood uplifting; improves digestion; improves mental clarity and memory

Cedarwood

Cedrus atlantica

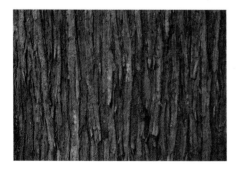

Scent: Woody

Uses

Reduces anxiety and tension; calming; relaxes tight muscles; helpful for meditation; lessens pain; promotes restful sleep; vapors help breathing; repels insects

Celery

Apium graveolens

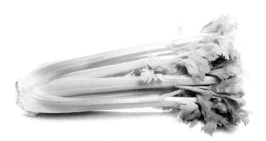

Scent: Strong celery

Uses

Reduces tension; calming; promotes restful sleep; helps reduce cellulite deposits; purifying effect on the body

Chamomile

Matricaria chamomilla and *Anthemis nobilis*

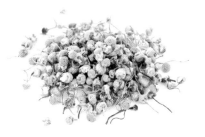

Scent: Musky

Uses

Reduces stress and tension; calming; lessens pain; promotes restful sleep; reduces inflammation; improves digestion; increases appetite; healing to the skin; soothes insect bites

Champaca Flower

Michelia alba, Michelia champaca

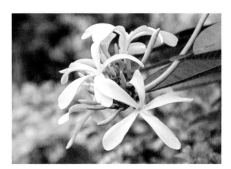

Scent: Floral

Uses

Warming to the body; reduces stress; calming; promotes a peaceful state; lifts up moods; euphoric; helps to breathe easier; fixative for perfumes and fragrances; deodorant

Cinnamon Bark and Leaf

Cinnamomum zeylanicum

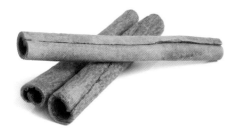

Scent: Cinnamon

Uses

Warming to the body; relaxes tight muscles; lessens pain; mood uplifting; aphrodisiac; helps relieve fatigue; improves digestion; increases appetite; helps reduce cellulite deposits; disinfectant; repels insects

Clary Sage

Salvia sclarea

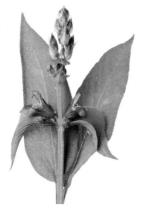

Scent: Sweet and spicy

Uses

Reduces stress and tension; calming; lessens pain; promotes restful sleep; aphrodisiac; improves digestion; contains estrogen-like hormone; encourages communication

Clove

Eugenia caryophyllata

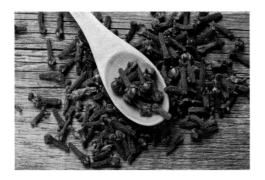

Scent: Hot and spicy

Uses

Warming to the body; relieves pain; mood uplifting; helps relieve fatigue; aphrodisiac; vapors help breathing; improves digestion; improves mental clarity and memory; disinfectant; repels insects

Coriander

Coriandrum sativum

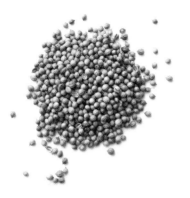

Scent: Musky

Uses

Relieves pain; helps relieve fatigue; Improves digestion; improves mental clarity and memory

Cubeb

Piper cubeba

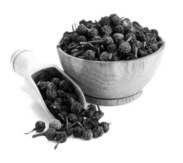

Scent: Peppery

Uses

Relieves pain; breaks up congestion; vapors help breathing; improves digestion

Cumin

Cuminum cyminum

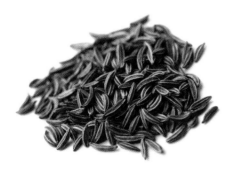

Scent: Strong spicy

Uses

Warming to the body; relieves pain; helps relieve fatigue; energizing; improves digestion

Cypress

Cupressus sempervirens

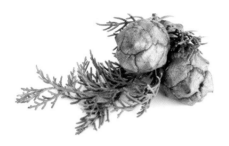

Scent: Woody

Uses

Reduces stress and tension; relaxes tight muscles; calming; promotes restful sleep; tegulates female reproductive system; teduces perspiration; helps reduce cellulite deposits; contracts weak connective tissue; tones skin; stops bleeding from injuries

Dill

Anethum graveolens

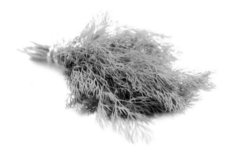

Scent: Spicy

Uses

Reduces stress; calming; relieves pain; promotes restful sleep; improves digestion; stimulates lactation in nursing mothers; repels insects

Elemi

Canarium commune,
Canarium luzonicum

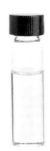

Scent: Lemony

Uses

Warming to the body; improves circulation; reduces stress; calming and relaxing; helpful for meditation; promotes restful sleep; lifts up moods; encourages communication of inner feelings; opens the breathing passages for deeper breathing; breaks up mucus (mild effect); healing to the skin; fixative for perfumes and fragrances

Eucalyptus

Eucalyptus globulus

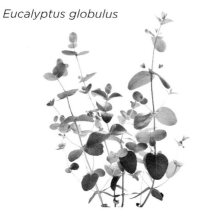

Scent: Fresh, camphorlike

Uses

Cooling to the body; relieves pain; refreshing; breaks up congestion; reduces inflammation; vapors help breathing; disinfectant; repels insects

Fennel

Foeniculum vulgare

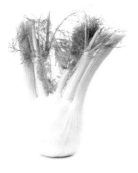

Scent: Strong licorice

Uses

Warming to the body; relieves pain; improves digestion; increases appetite; contains estrogen-like hormone; stimulates lactation in nursing mothers; helps reduce cellulite deposits; purifying effect on the body; repels insects

Frankincense

Boswellia thurifera

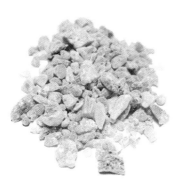

Scent: Woody and camphorlike

Uses

Calming; helpful for meditation; promotes restful sleep; reduces inflammation; encourages communication; healing to the skin and wrinkles

Geranium

Pelargonium graveolens

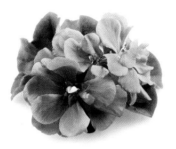

Scent: Roselike

Uses

Reduces stress and tension; calming in small amounts; stimulating in large amounts; lessens pain; mood uplifting; reduces inflammation; encourages communication; helps reduce cellulite deposits; stops bleeding from injuries; soothes itching skin; repels insects

Ginger

Zingiber officinale

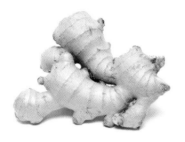

Scent: Spicy

Uses

Warming to the body; relaxes tight muscles; relieves pain; mood uplifting; aphrodisiac; helps relieve fatigue; energizing; improves digestion; increases appetite; improves mental clarity and memory

Grapefruit

Citrus paradisi

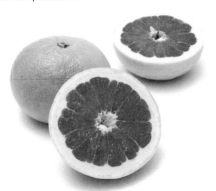

Scent: Citrus

Uses

Cooling to the body; mood uplifting; helps relieve fatigue; refreshing; energizing; increases physical strength; improves mental clarity and memory; helps reduce cellulite deposits; purifying effect on the body

Guaiacwood

*Bulnesia sarmienti,
Guaiacum officinale*

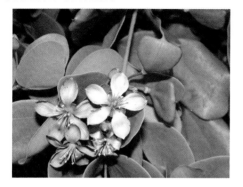

Scent: Sweet woody

Uses

Reduces stress and tension; calming and relaxing; helpful for meditation; relaxes tight muscles; promotes restful sleep; mood uplifting; reduces inflammation; soothes swollen and injured skin tissue; improves mental clarity; purifying to the tissues; soothes insect bites; relieves itching; fixative for perfumes and fragrances

Jasmine

Jasminum officinale

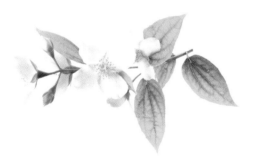

Scent: Sweet floral

Uses

Mood uplifting; aphrodisiac

Juniper Berries

Juniperus communis

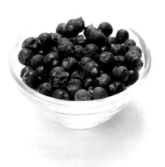

Scent: Evergreen forest

Uses

Lessens pain; energizing; reduces inflammation; improves mental clarity and memory; helps reduce cellulite deposits; purifying to the body; soothes insect bites; repels insects

Lavender

Lavandula officinalis

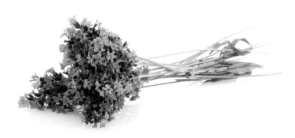

Scent: Fresh and clean

Uses

Reduces stress and tension; calming in small amounts; stimulating in large amounts; relaxes tight muscles; lessens pain; promotes restful sleep; mood uplifting; balances mood swings; breaks up congestion; reduces inflammation; vapors help breathing; improves digestion; purifying to the body; disinfectant; healing to the skin; soothes insect bites; repels insects

Lemon

Citrus limonum

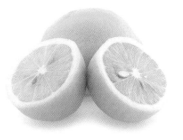

Scent: Lemony

Uses

Cooling to the body; balancing, calming, or energizing; balances nervous system; mood uplifting; helps relieve fatigue; refreshing; improves mental clarity and memory; helps reduce cellulite deposits; purifying effect on the body; stops bleeding from injuries; disinfectant; soothes insect bites

Lemongrass

Cymbopogon citratus

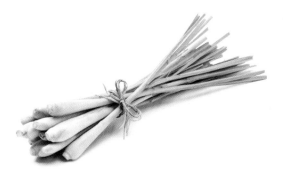

Scent: Strong lemon

Uses

Calming; balances nervous system; mood uplifting; reduces inflammation; vapors help breathing; improves digestion; stimulates lactation in nursing mothers; contracts weak connective tissue; disinfectant; tones skin; repels insects

Lime

Citrus limetta

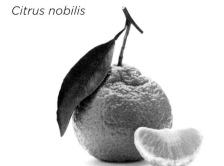

Scent: Fresh citrus

Uses

Cooling to the body; mood uplifting; helps relieve fatigue; refreshing; energizing; improves mental clarity and memory; helps reduce cellulite deposits; purifying effect on the body; disinfectant; soothes insect bites

Mandarin

Citrus nobilis

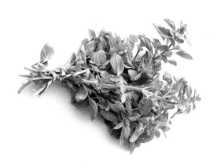

Scent: Sweet citrus

Uses

Cooling to the body; reduces stress and tension; calming; mood uplifting

Marjoram

Origanum marjorana

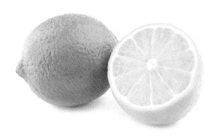

Scent: Sweet and spicy

Uses

Warming to the body; calming; relaxes tight muscles; promotes restful sleep; breaks up congestion; reduces inflammation; vapors help breathing; improves digestion; disinfectant; soothes insect bites

Melissa

Melissa officinalis

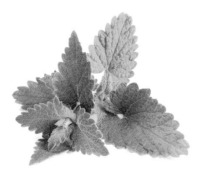

Scent: Lemony

Uses

Reduces stress and anxiety; calming and relaxing; relieves aches and pains; promotes restful sleep; mood uplifting

Myrrh

Commiphora myrrha

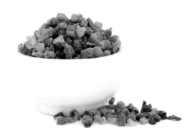

Scent: Bitter

Uses

Helpful for meditation; mood uplifting; reduces inflammation; healing to the skin

Myrtle

Myrtus communis

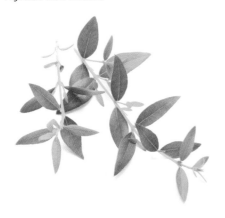

Scent: Fresh, camphorlike

Uses

Calming; vapors help breathing

Neroli

Citrus aurantium

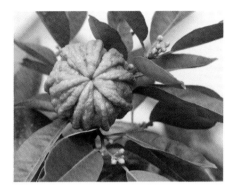

Scent: Sweet floral

Uses

Relieves nervous tension; promotes restful sleep; mood uplifting

---

Nutmeg

Myristica fragrans

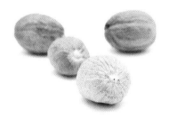

Scent: Spicy

Uses

Calming in small amounts; stimulating in large amounts; relaxes tight muscles; relieves pain; improves digestion

---

Orange

Citrus aurantium

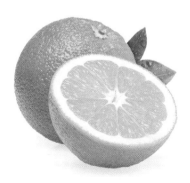

Scent: Sweet orange

Uses

Cooling to the body; reduces stress; calming; promotes restful sleep; mood uplifting; purifying effect on the body

Palmarosa

Cymbopogon martini

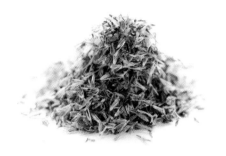

Scent: Sweet

Uses

Warming to the body; relaxes tight muscles; lessens pain; mood uplifting; reduces inflammation; healing, regenerating, moisturizing for skin

---

Patchouli

Pogostemon patchouli

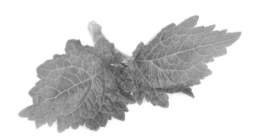

Scent: Musky

Uses

Mood uplifting; aphrodisiac; nerve stimulant; disinfectant; healing to the skin; repels insects

---

Black Pepper

Piper nigrum

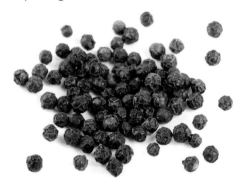

Scent: Hot and spicy

Uses

Warming to the body; relaxes tight muscles; improves digestion

Peppermint

Mentha piperita

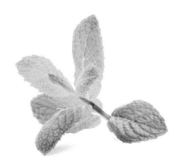

Scent: Strong mint

Uses

Cooling to the body; relieves pain; mood uplifting; helps relieve fatigue; aphrodisiac; refreshing; energizing; nerve stimulant; increases physical strength; breaks up congestion; reduces inflammation; vapors help breathing; improves digestion; increases appetite; reduces lactation in nursing mothers; improves mental clarity and memory; soothes itching skin; repels insects

Peru Balsam

Myroxylon pereirae

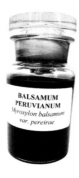

Scent: Vanilla

Uses

Warming to the body; calming; promotes restful sleep; mood uplifting; healing to the skin

Petitgrain

Citrus bigarade

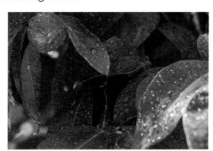

Scent: Slightly citrus

Uses

Reduces anxiety, stress, and tension; calming; promotes restful sleep; mood uplifting; improves mental clarity and memory; healing to the skin

Pine

Pinus sylvestris

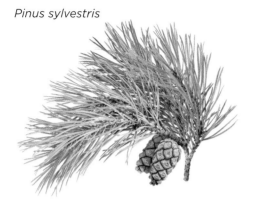

Scent: Fresh pine

Uses

Lessens pain; mood uplifting; helps relieve fatigue; refreshing; energizing; increases physical strength; breaks up congestion; vapors help breathing; improves mental clarity and memory; purifying effect on the body; disinfectant

Rose

Rosa centifolia and *Rosa damascena*

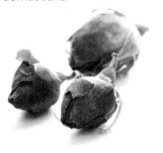

Scent: Rosy

Uses

Calming; lessens pain; mood uplifting; aphrodisiac; increases physical strength; reduces inflammation; purifying effect on the body; healing to the skin

Rosemary

Rosmarinus officinalis

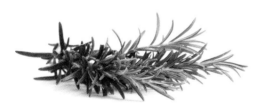

Scent: Strong camphor

Uses

Relaxes tight muscles; relieves pain; mood uplifting; helps relieve fatigue; energizing; nerve stimulant; vapors help breathing; improves digestion; improves mental clarity and memory; helps reduce cellulite deposits; purifying effect on the body; disinfectant; repels insects

Sage

Salvia officinalis

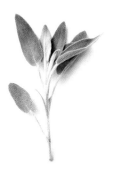

Scent: Spicy

Uses

Lessens pain; reduces lactation in nursing mothers; reduces perspiration; purifying effect on the body; disinfectant

Sandalwood

Santalum album

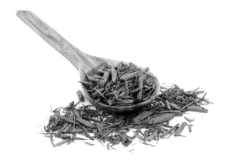

Scent: Woody

Uses

Reduces stress; calming; helpful for meditation; promotes restful sleep; mood uplifting; aphrodisiac; healing to the skin

Spearmint

Mentha spicata

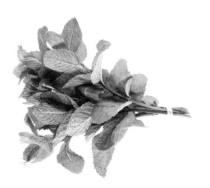

Scent: Minty

Uses

Cooling to the body; relieves pain; mood uplifting; helps relieve fatigue; aphrodisiac; refreshing; energizing; nerve stimulant; increases physical strength; breaks up congestion; reduces inflammation; vapors help breathing; improves digestion; increases appetite; improves mental clarity and memory; soothes itching skin; repels insects

Spikenard

Nardostachys grandiflora,
Nardostachys jatamansi

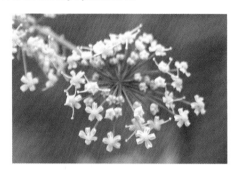

Scent: Earthy

Uses

Reduces stress; calming; promotes restful sleep; mood uplifting; reduces inflammation; fixative for perfumes and fragrances; deodorant

Spruce

Picea mariana

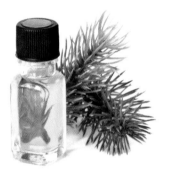

Scent: Sweet pinelike

Uses

Calming; breaks up congestion; vapors help breathing; encourages communication

Tea Tree

Melaleuca alternifolia

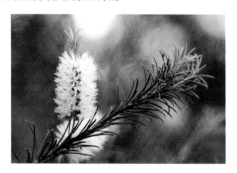

Scent: Camphorlike

Uses

Lessens pain; vapors help breathing; disinfectant; healing to the skin

Thyme

Thymus vulgaris

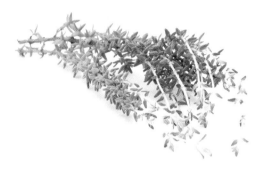

Scent: Hot and spicy

Uses

Warming to the body; relaxes tight muscles; lessens pain; mood uplifting; aphrodisiac; increases physical strength; breaks up congestion; reduces inflammation; vapors help breathing; improves digestion; increases appetite; increases perspiration; improves mental clarity and memory; helps reduce cellulite deposits; purifying effect on the body; disinfectant; repels insects

Tolu Balsam

Myroxlon toluiferum

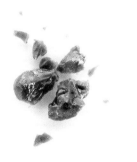

Scent: Floral

Uses

Mood uplifting; fixative for perfumes and fragrances; deodorant

Vanilla CO_2 extract

Vanilla fragrans, Vanilla planifolia

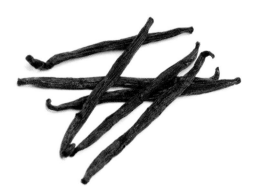

Scent: Sweet

Uses

Reduces stress; calming; promotes restful sleep; encourages dreaming; mood uplifting; aphrodisiac; fixative for perfumes and fragrances; deodorant

Vetiver

Vetiveria zizanoides

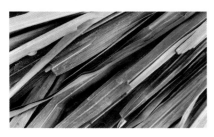

Scent: Earthy

Uses

Reduces stress and tension; calming; relaxes tight muscles; relieves pain; promotes restful sleep; increases physical strength; healing to the skin; repels insects

Ylang-Ylang

Cananga odorata

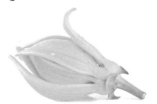

Scent: Sweet floral

Uses

Calming; relaxes tight muscles; lessens pain; promotes restful sleep; mood uplifting; aphrodisiac; encourages communication; disinfectant

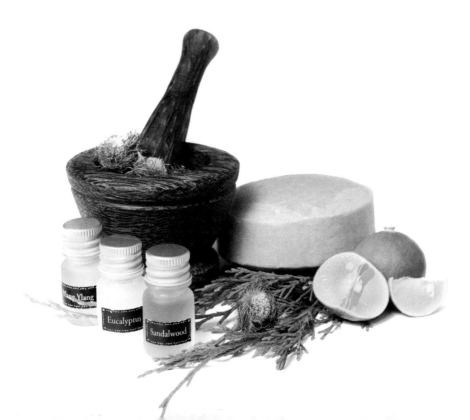

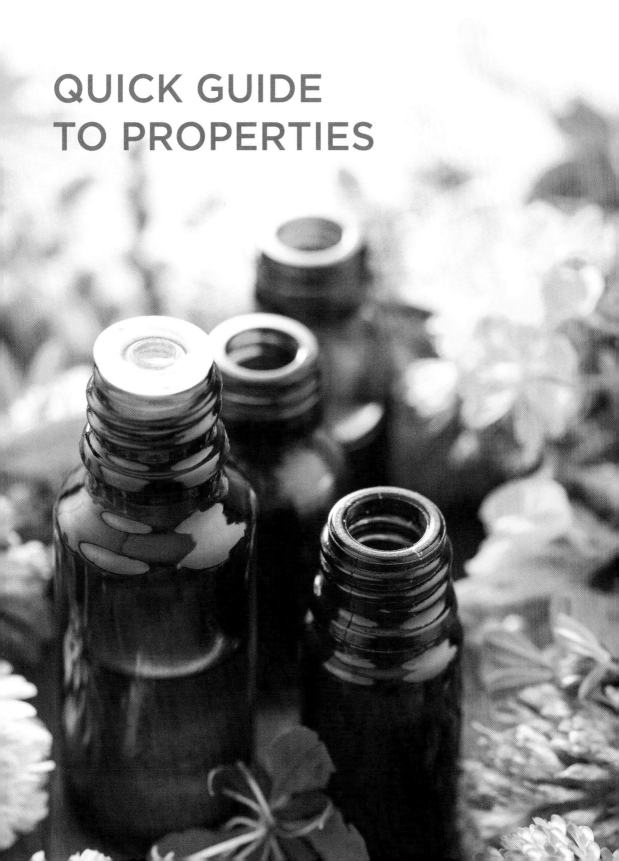

QUICK GUIDE
TO PROPERTIES

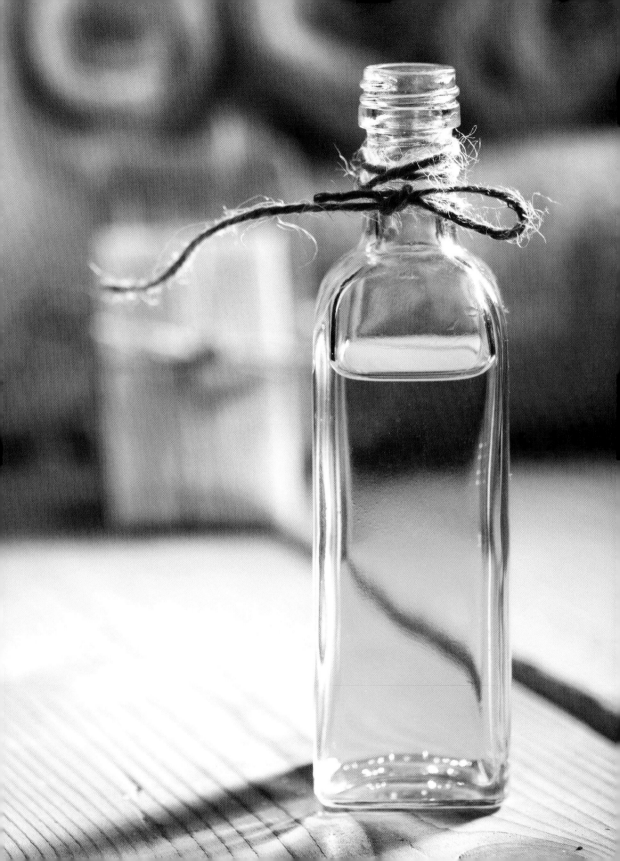

Aphrodisiac

Anise, clary sage, cinnamon, clove, ginger, jasmine, patchouli, peppermint, rose, sandalwood, spearmint, thyme, vanilla CO_2, ylang-ylang

Appetite (Increases)

Anise, caraway, chamomile, cinnamon, fennel, ginger, peppermint, spearmint, thyme

Bleeding (To stop)

Cypress, geranium, lemon

Breathing

Allspice, anise, (sweet) bay, cajeput, caraway, cedarwood, champaca flower, clove, cubeb, elemi, eucalyptus, guaicwood, lavender, lemongrass, marjoram, myrtle, peppermint, pine, rosemary, spearmint, spruce, tea tree, thyme, vanilla CO_2

Calming

Allspice, anise, (sweet) basil, (sweet) bay, benzoin, bois de rose, cajeput, cedarwood, celery, chamomile, clary sage, cypress, dill, frankincense, geranium, lavender, lemon, lemongrass, mandarin, marjoram, melissa, myrtle, nutmeg, orange, Peru balsam, petitgrain, rose, sandalwood, spikenard, spruce, vetiver, ylang-ylang

Cellulite

(Sweet) basil, benzoin, celery, cinnamon, cypress, fennel, geranium, grapefruit, juniper berries, lemon, lime, rosemary, thyme

Communication (Encourages)

Clary sage, elemi, frankincense, geranium, spruce, ylang-ylang

Congestion

Benzoin, cajeput, cubeb, elemi, eucalyptus, lavender, marjoram, peppermint, pine, spearmint, spruce, thyme

Connective Tissue (Tightens)

Cypress, lemongrass

Cooling

Eucalyptus, grapefruit, lemon, lime, mandarin, orange, peppermint, spearmint

Deodorant

Champaca flower, spikenard, tolu balsam, vanilla CO_2

Digestion

Allspice, anise, (sweet) basil, (sweet) bay, caraway, cardamom, chamomile, cinnamon, clary sage, clove, coriander, cubeb, cumin, dill, fennel, ginger, lavender, lemongrass, marjoram, nutmeg, black pepper, peppermint, rosemary, spearmint, thyme

Disinfectant

Allspice, (sweet) bay, bergamot, cajeput, cinnamon, clove, eucalyptus, lavender, lemon, lemongrass, lime, marjoram, patchouli, pine, rosemary, sage, tea tree, thyme, ylang-ylang

Energizing

Cumin, ginger, grapefruit, juniper berries, lemon, lime, peppermint, pine, rosemary, spearmint

Fatigue (Relieves)

(Sweet) basil, bergamot, cinnamon, clove, coriander, cumin, ginger, grapefruit, lemon, lime, peppermint, pine, rosemary, spearmint

Female Reproductive System Regulator

Clary sage, cypress, fennel

Fixative

Benzoin, champaca flower, elemi, guaiacwood, patchouli, sandalwood, spikenard, tolu balsam, vanilla CO_2

Inflammation

Benzoin, chamomile, eucalyptus, guaiacwood, frankincense, geranium, juniper berries, lavender, lemongrass, marjoram, myrrh, palmarosa, peppermint, rose, spearmint, spikenard, thyme

Insect Bites

(Sweet) basil, chamomile, guaiacwood, juniper berries, lavender, lemon, lime, marjoram

Insect Repellent

(Sweet) bay, cajeput, cedarwood, cinnamon, clove, dill, eucalyptus, fennel, geranium, lavender, lemongrass, patchouli, peppermint, rosemary, spearmint, thyme, vetiver

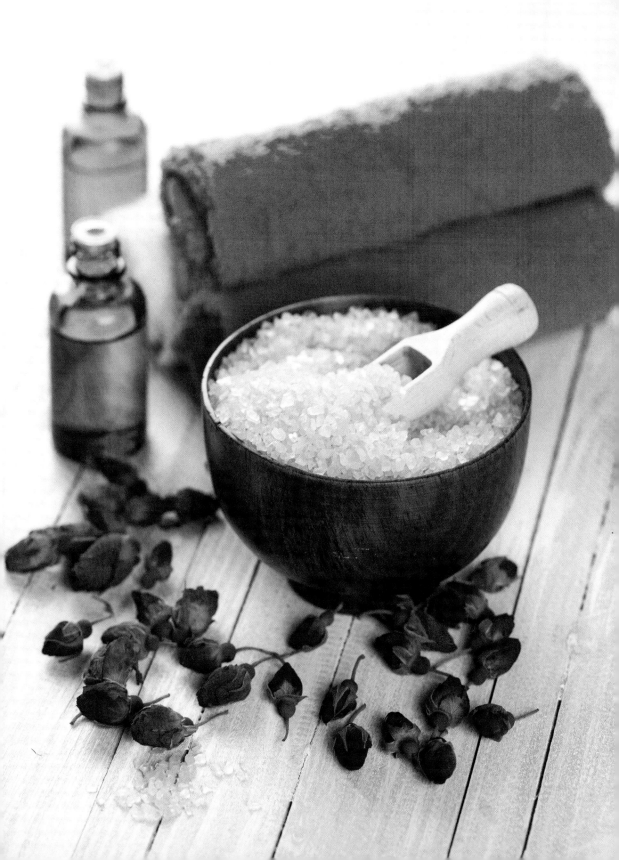

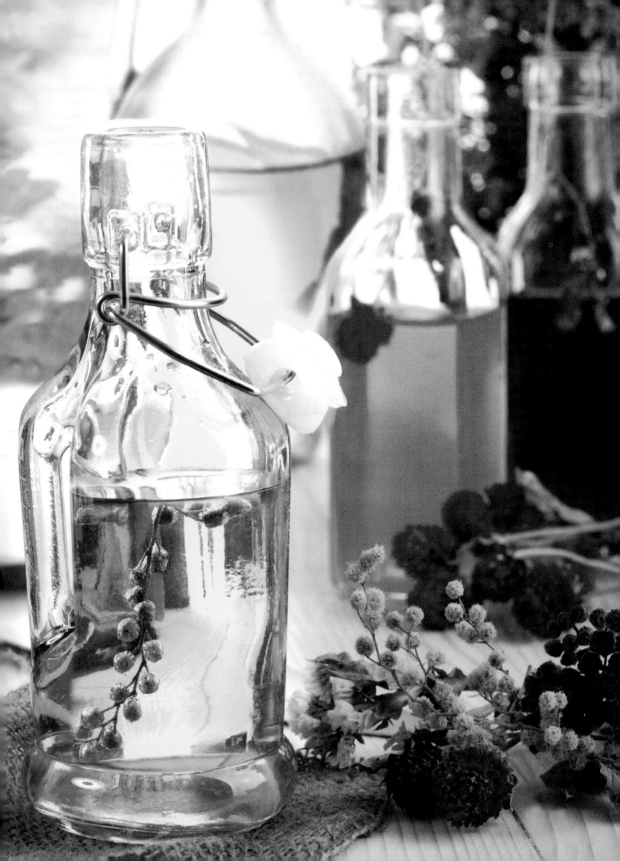

Lactation

(To decrease) Peppermint, sage

(To increase) Anise, (sweet) basil, caraway, dill, fennel, lemongrass

Meditation

Benzoin, cedarwood, elemi, frankincense, guaiacwood, myrrh, sandalwood

Mental Clarity and Memory Improvement

(Sweet) basil, (sweet) bay, cardamom, clove, coriander, ginger, guaiacwood, grapefruit, juniper berries, lemon, lime, peppermint, petitgrain, rosemary, spearmint, thyme

Moisturizing

Aloe, bois de rose, palmarosa

Mood Swings

Lavender

Mood Uplifting

Allspice, (sweet) basil, benzoin, bergamot, bois de rose, cardamom, champaca flower, cinnamon, clove, elemi, geranium, ginger, grapefruit, guaiacwood, jasmine, lavender, lemon, lemongrass, lime, mandarin, melissa, myrrh, neroli, orange, palmarosa, patchouli, peppermint, Peru balsam, petitgrain, pine, rose, rosemary, sandalwood, spearmint, spikenard, thyme, tolu balsam, vanilla CO_2, ylang-ylang

Muscle Tension Relief

Allspice, (sweet) bay, benzoin, cajeput, cedarwood, cinnamon, cypress, ginger, lavender, nutmeg, palmarosa, black pepper, rosemary, thyme, vetiver

Nerve Stimulant

Patchouli, peppermint, rosemary, spearmint

Nervous System (Balancing)

Bergamot, lemon, lemongrass

Pain

Allspice, anise, (sweet) basil, (sweet) bay, bois de rose, cajeput, caraway, cardamom, cedarwood, chamomile, cinnamon, clary sage, clove, coriander, cubeb, cumin, dill, eucalyptus, fennel, geranium, ginger, juniper berries, lavender, melissa, nutmeg, palmarosa, peppermint, pine, rose, rosemary, sage, spearmint, tea tree, thyme, vetiver, ylang-ylang

Physical Endurance

Grapefruit, peppermint, pine, rose, spearmint, thyme, vetiver

Perspiration (Increases)

(Sweet) bay, thyme (Reduces) Cypress, sage

Purifying

(Sweet) basil, celery, fennel, grapefruit, guaiacwood, juniper berries, lavender, lemon, lime, orange, pine, rose, rosemary, sage, thyme

Refreshing

Eucalyptus, grapefruit, lemon, lime, peppermint, pine, spearmint

Skin Care

Aloe, benzoin, bois de rose, chamomile, elemi, frankincense, lavender, myrrh, palmarosa, patchouli, Peru balsam, petitgrain, rose, sandalwood, tea tree, vetiver

Skin (Stops itching)

Geranium, guaiacwood, peppermint, Peru balsam, spearmint

Skin Toning

Cypress, lemongrass

Sleep Restfully

Allspice, anise, (sweet) basil, (sweet) bay, benzoin, bois de rose, cajeput, cedarwood, celery, chamomile, clary sage, cypress, dill, elemi, frankincense, guaiacwood, lavender, marjoram, melissa, neroli, orange, Peru balsam, petitgrain, sandalwood, spikenard, vanilla CO_2, vetiver, ylang-ylang

Stress Relief

Allspice, benzoin, bergamot, bois de rose, cedarwood, celery, chamomile, champaca flower, clary sage, cypress, dill, elemi, geranium, guaiacwood, lavender, mandarin, melissa, orange, petitgrain, sandalwood, spikenard, vanilla CO_2, vetiver

Warming

Allspice, benzoin, cajeput, cardamom, champaca flower, cinnamon, clove, cumin, elemi, fennel, ginger, marjoram, palmarosa, black pepper, Peru balsam, thyme

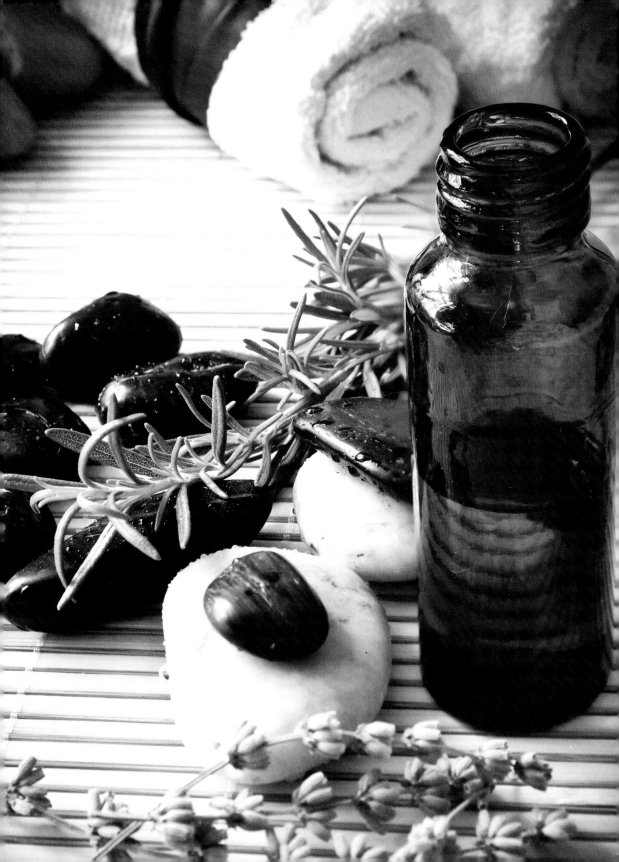

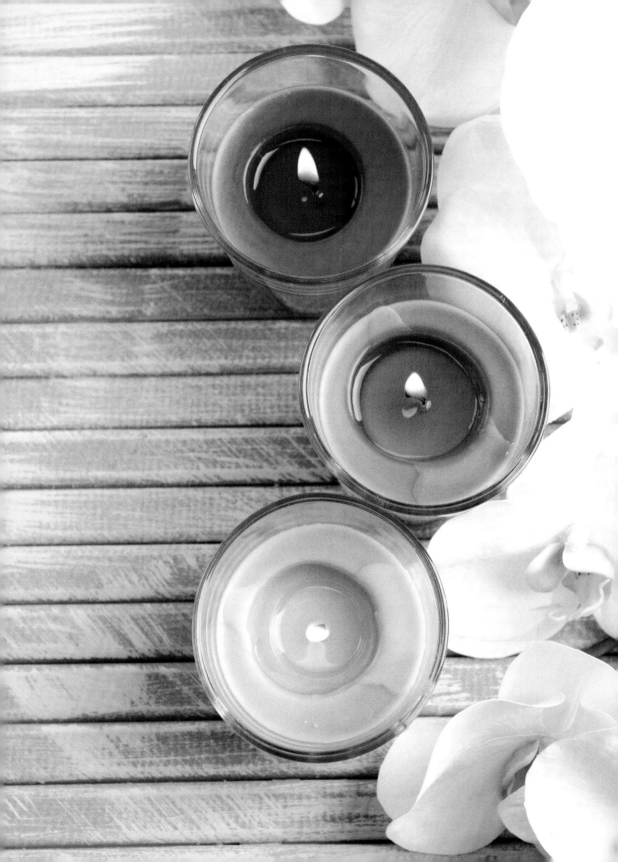

Index

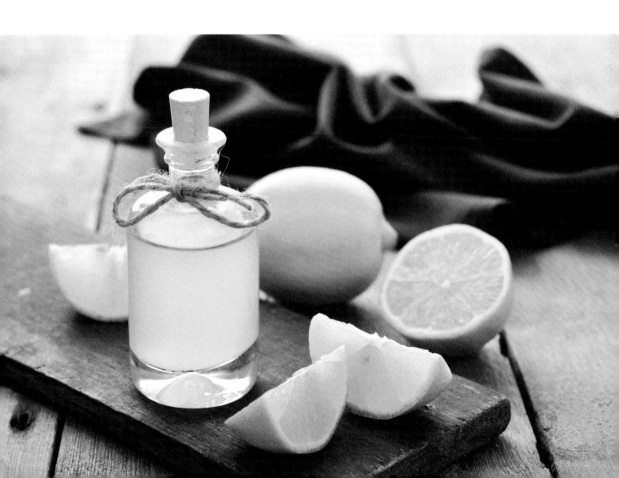

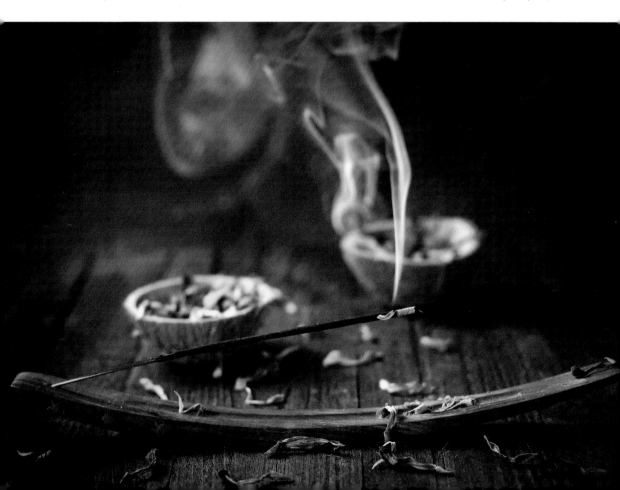

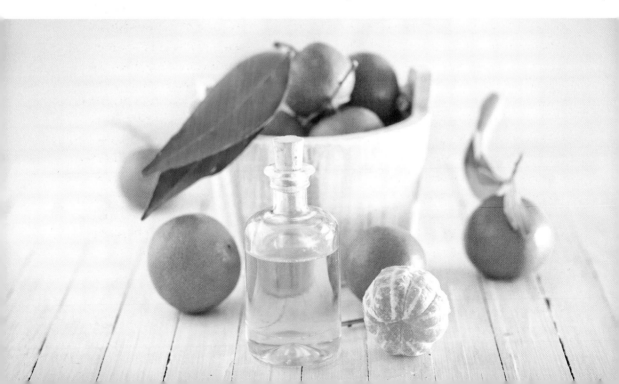

Photo Credits

Courtesy Wikimedia Foundation/Itineranttrader: 158 (bottom); Forest & Kim Starr, 161 (top); Maša Sinreih in Valentina Vivod 167 (middle), 171 (middle)

Istockphoto: © ALLEKO 85, 156 (middle); © Christopher Ames 147 (bottom); © Angie Photos 161 (bottom); © Apixelintime 134, 154 (middle); © Avalon Studio 81, 108; © belchonock 145 (grapeseed), 182; © Bienchen-s 168 (bottom); © Botamochi 46; © Burwellphotography 145 (flaxseed); © Creativeye99 113, 152 (top); © Daffodilred 60, 177; © Dionisvero 151 (middle); © Dkgilbey 31; © Dulezidar 71, 73; © Kevin Dyer 147 (middle); © Elenathewise 155 (middle); © Chris Elwell 66; © Fcw 152 (bottom); © Keith Ferris Photo 151 (bottom); © Floortje 123, 152 (middle), 157 (bottom), 163 (bottom), 169 (top); © Fotostorm 18–19; © Gojak 72; Andrey Gorulko 157 (middle); © Gvictoria 53; © Hohenhaus 76; © Hiorgos 56; © Oliver Hoffmann 144 (middle); © Hudiemm 91, 160 (middle); © IvonneW 162 (top); © Gabor Izso 157 (bottom); © Silvia Jansen 104, 144 (bottom); © Anna Kucherova 168 (top); © Kyoshino 154 (bottom); © Lepas2004 105, 169 (bottom); © Niki Litov 174; © Loooby 89; © Loops7 158 (middle); © Lujing 162 (middle); © Luknaja 172 (top); © Marilyna 40, 190–191; © Marrakeshh 115; © Mashuk 55, 145 (jojoba), 163 (middle), 167 (top); © Matejay 146 (macadamia); © Mikolette 5; © Olga Miltsova 8; © Miss J 10–11, 32; © Marek Mnich 124, 156 (top); © Narcisa 147 (top); © Ockra 166 (bottom); © Okea 162 (bottom); © Olgaorly 148–149; © Frank Oppermann 171 (bottom); © Phadungsakphoto 153 (top); © Pjohnson1 159 (middle); © Popovaphoto 158 (top); © Sasha Radosavljevic 49, 156 (bottom); © Rafcha 146 (kukui); © Ranplett 155 (top); © RedHelga 165 (bottom); © Dirk Richter 159 (bottom): © Smuay 24; © Suprunvitaly 144 (top); © Synergee 22, 168 (middle); © Tashka2000 185; © Tycoon751 20, 188; © Alina Solovyova-Vincent 102, 151; © Vinodkumarm 155 (bottom); © Matka Wariatka 39, 57, 121, 128, 130, 139, 145 (hazelnut); © Michael Westhoff 12; Chamille White 150; Zeljkosantrac 178

Shutterstock: © AS Food Studio 47; © Marilyn Barbone 169 (middle); © Katarina Christenson 170 (bottom); © Dionisvera 163 (top); © Drozdowski 171 (top); © Epitavi 36, 170 (middle); © Foodpictures 69; Fotohunter 42–43; © Happydancing 52; © Haraldmuc 167 (bottom); © Image Point Fr 34; © JPC-PROD 59, 99; © Malgorzata Kistryn 165 (top); © KPG Payless2 159 (top); © Tamara Kulikova 165 (middle); © Charlotte Lake 64, 154 (top); © Leonardo Da 26, 96; © Madlen 82; © Olga Miltsova 17, 173; © Nenov Brothers Images 160 (top); © Piccia Neri 181; © Nookieme 83; © Olesia 172 (bottom); © Optimarc 153 (middle); © Pittaya 172 (middle); © Praisaeng 62; © Pressmaster 6–7; Rido 146 (olive); © Rickyd 153 (bottom); © Sea Wave 41, 142–143, 146 (sesame); © Spline X 101; © Sripfoto 14–15; © Alex Staroseltsev 126, 160 (bottom); © Sunny Forest 186; © TGTGTG 58; © Vesna 48; Valentyn Volkov 161 (middle); © Wasanajai 166 (middle); © ZIGROUP-CREATIONS 166 (top)

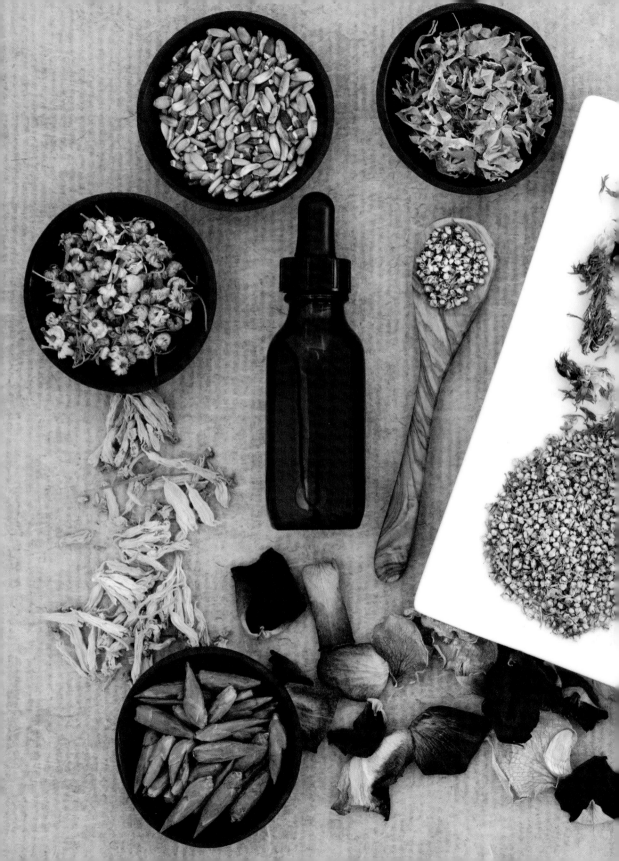

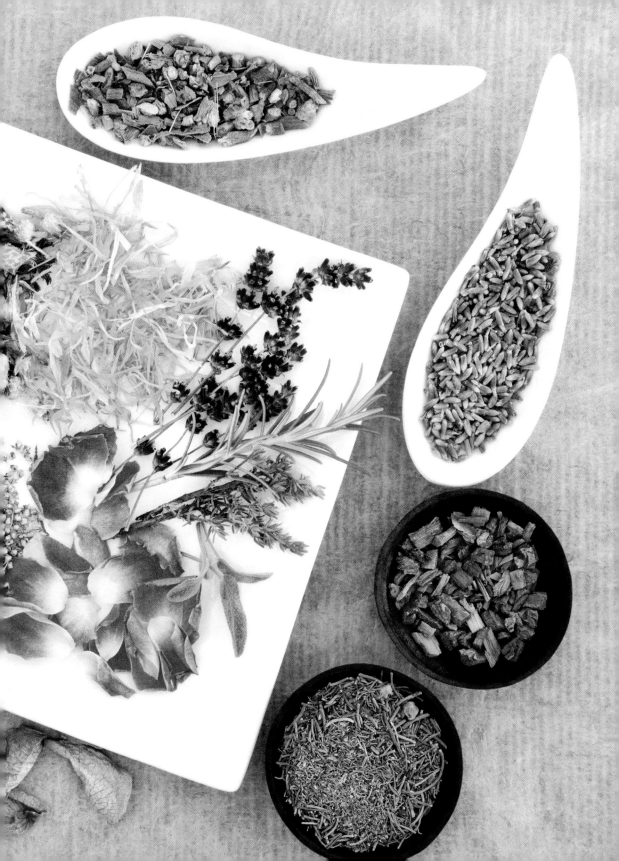

About the Authors

Carol Schiller and David Schiller are the authors of seven published books on the use of essential oils. Since 1986, Carol and David have studied and researched the benefits of plant oils, and determining their practical uses and applications. They have been instructing classes and training workshops for companies, colleges, and other educational organizations since 1989. Carol has been a featured presenter at international conferences.